YOU CAN BUT YOU DON'T WANT TO.

IF YOU WANT TO, YOU CAN.

PRINCIPLES THAT WILL CHANGE YOUR GAME

SHAH EMRAN

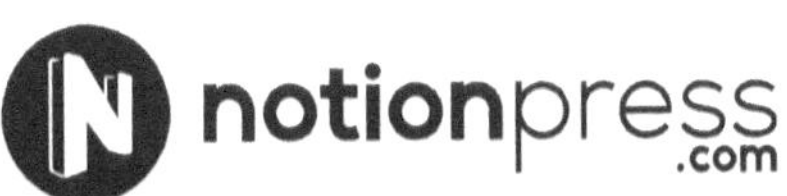

INDIA · SINGAPORE · MALAYSIA

ISBN
Paperback 979-8-89673-346-1
Hardcase 979-8-89777-662-7

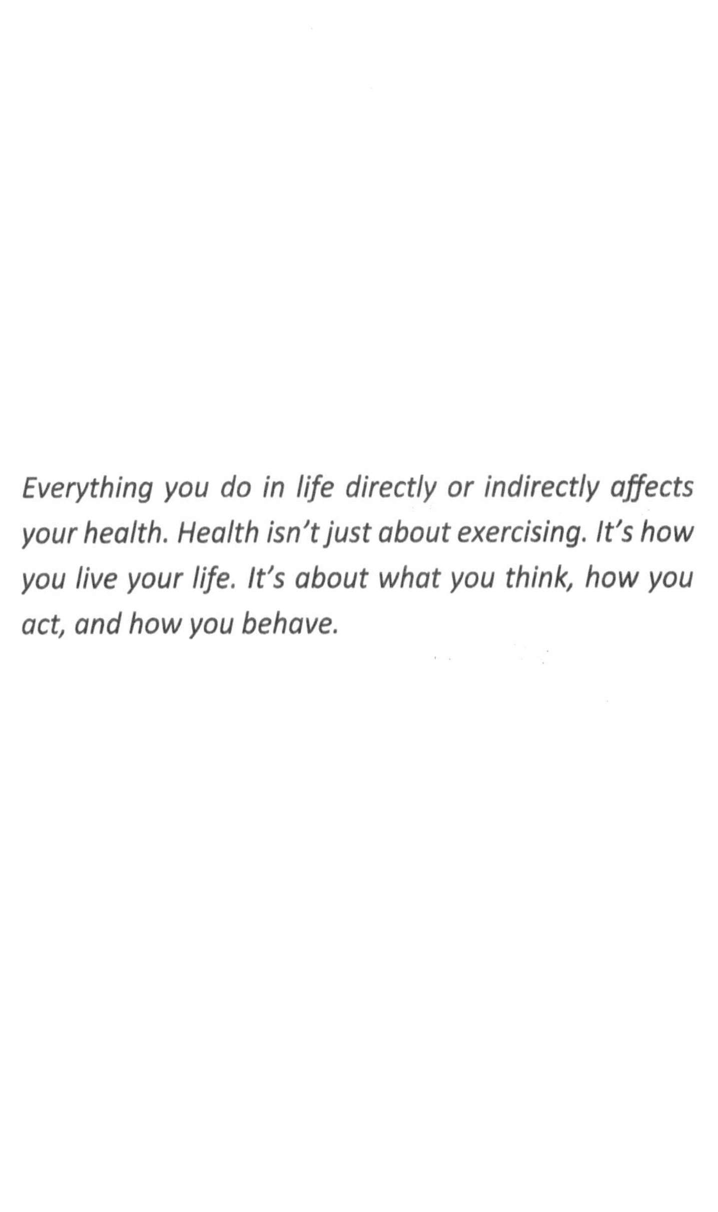

Everything you do in life directly or indirectly affects your health. Health isn't just about exercising. It's how you live your life. It's about what you think, how you act, and how you behave.

The best advice I can give you is to accept and love yourself fully and do it without any excuses.

Contents

Let's Have Some Dessert, Shall We?

One evening, I was invited to a friend's place for dinner. After a delicious meal, she served a warm, tempting custard. "Let's have some dessert, shall we?" she said with a smile. My mouth watered just looking at it! My friend's husband, though, seemed surprised. "Shah won't eat that," he said. "He's very health-conscious."

Now, I take care of my health, but depriving myself of life's little pleasures? Absolutely not! I dished myself a generous portion of that yummy custard. My friend's husband was quite amazed. Here I was, this health nut, enjoying a dessert full of sugar.

Later that night, he came up to me and said, "Shah, how do you do it?"

"Do what?" I asked.

"Eat all this food and still stay healthy and fit," he said.

We ended up talking for a long time that night. One of the biggest hurdles people face is the fear of giving up their favourite foods. But here's the thing: a healthy lifestyle doesn't mean saying goodbye to everything you enjoy. It's about finding balance.

And that's when it hit me that there are many people out there, just like my friend, people who think being healthy means saying goodbye to their favourite foods and spending hours sweating it out at the gym.

That night, I decided I wanted to share something with the world. Health isn't a complicated mystery we've made it out to be. It's about feeling good and living a life that's truly satisfying.

This book is my way of helping people like my friend. It's about showing that healthy living isn't a punishment; it's a path to happiness and a more fulfilling life.

Since you've opened this book, I'm guessing you're someone who wants to learn, grow, and live a life that's both happy and healthy. That's fantastic! Consider me your personal trainer on this journey.

I'll be your trainer, but instead of barbells, we'll be using knowledge and experiences; instead of muscles, we'll be working on your overall well-being. I'll be here with you every step of the way, sharing everything I've witnessed and experienced, everything I've learned and unlearned. That's right, even the things I learned weren't always helpful, and sometimes we need to 'unlearn' them. I'll share all I've seen and done in the hopes that it helps you on your own path. We'll learn together, unpacking old ideas and discovering new ones.

There will be challenges, of course. But that's okay! Challenges are how we grow. Nobody gets it perfect all the time. The important thing is to keep moving forward, one step at a time.

This book won't be filled with complicated words or hard-to-follow advice. We'll keep things simple and clear, focusing on practical things that you can use in your everyday life. Whether it's about healthy habits, reaching your goals, or feeling good about yourself, we'll tackle it together.

Growth and learning are lifelong journeys, and there's always something new to discover. With a bit of effort and this book as your companion, you'll be well on your way to a happy and healthy life. So, get comfortable, turn the page, and let's begin this adventure together.

Building a Community of Wellness Together

Have you ever felt that spark – the joy of watching someone light up as they discover their own path to a healthier, happier life? That's the magic I'm chasing. As a fitness fanatic who's already on this incredible journey, I get to share my knowledge, experiences, and everything I've learned with others. Why? Because I want to see YOU take charge of your well-being and become the strongest, most awesome version of yourself.

The thing is that there's no one-size-fits-all plan for health. We're all unique, with our own goals, challenges, and situations. That's why empathy, understanding, and zero judgement are key.

The best way to inspire someone is to lead by example. When I prioritise my own health and well-being, I'm showing you that positive changes are possible, and the results can stick! Sharing my triumphs, struggles, and everything in-between isn't about bragging – it's about offering real-life insights and encouragement, especially when you're feeling overwhelmed. My hope is that my honesty will inspire you to take that first step towards a life that's healthier and more fulfilling.

But it's not just about inspiration. I want to equip you with the tools and resources you need to win on your path to optimal health and success. By giving you the knowledge and skills to make informed decisions and take action towards your goals, I'm empowering you to become the boss of your own well-being.

Inspiring people to chase health and success is a gift that keeps on giving. It can truly change lives, and not just yours. By sharing my passion, knowledge, and experiences, I want to create a ripple effect of positive change, a wave that reaches far beyond myself. Imagine a community where everyone supports, encourages, and empowers each other to reach their full potential and live their best life. That's the kind of world I want to build, and that's why I'm writing this book – to help you achieve your health goals and join the movement.

If I Can Do It, You Can Do It Too

I don't drive an expensive car or live in a huge bungalow. I do not own a Rolex, nor do I have a million dollars in my bank account. But I do have time and energy to spend with myself and my loved ones. I live a joyful, healthy life.

Things get better if you think better.

True happiness doesn't come with a price tag. It's brewed in the quiet moments, the connections with loved ones, and the simple joy of living a healthy life. This book isn't a magic spell promising instant transformation. It's a collection of lessons I've learned, a roadmap I've followed to reach my own happy and healthy haven.

If you're searching for a quick fix, this book might disappoint. But if you're willing to walk the path to make small changes that lead to big results, then keep reading. Because trust me, if I can do it, you can do it too.

This book isn't about bragging about my simple, happy, and healthy life. It's about sharing the tools that helped me build it. Maybe you won't wear a Rolex or live in a mansion either, but you can have fulfilling relationships, a healthy body, and a heart brimming with joy. Sound good? Let's dive in.

As you turn the pages, picture yourself living a life that feels good from the inside out. Imagine waking up with a sense of purpose, your body fuelled by healthy choices, and your heart connected to loved ones. That's the kind of happiness we're chasing here.

While you're reading through these pages, you might find yourself saying, "Hey, that's me!" I do this all the time, too. That's the whole point, isn't it? To learn, to grow, and to do things better. Even if you think you're doing something right, there's always more to learn. People can only change and improve if they know their mistakes. How can you get better if you don't even know what you're doing wrong?

Let's ditch the fantasy of a million-dollar life and build a reality that's rich in meaning, health, connection, and joy.

1

Wake-up Call

You know the feeling, that delicious wave of relief after solving a problem. You unclogged a drain, finished a tough project, or finally figured out that tricky recipe. Problems, though annoying, can be strangely satisfying to overcome. But what about a problem that whispers instead of shouts, a problem that hides in plain sight – our health?

Many people don't see their health as a problem until it becomes one.

Many people don't see their health as a problem until it becomes one. They feel 'fine', but 'fine' doesn't always mean healthy. You are driving down a sunny highway, windows down, music playing. Life feels good. Suddenly, a glaring orange light appears on your dashboard: the check engine light. Panic sets in. Is it something major? Should you pull over? Maybe it'll go away if you ignore it.

Our health is a lot like that check engine light. It sends us subtle (and sometimes not-so-subtle) signals, but often, we ignore them. We feel a bit sluggish, have trouble sleeping, or experience some aches and pains. But because these problems don't feel urgent or life-threatening, we brush them off, hoping they'll disappear. Just like a neglected check engine light can lead to serious car trouble, ignoring our health has significant consequences down the road. Just like a car running a little rough, our bodies show subtle signs that things aren't quite right.

Your health is your most valuable asset.

There's a saying, "An ounce of prevention is worth a pound of cure." By seeing subtle health issues as problems to address, you can take proactive steps to prevent them from becoming bigger problems down the road.

Taking care of your health doesn't require drastic changes overnight. It's about making small, sustainable improvements to your daily routine.

When you take care of your health, you have more energy to do the things you love. Whether it's playing with your kids, chasing after your dreams, or simply enjoying a good book, feeling good physically, mentally, and emotionally allows you to live life to the fullest. Sometimes, we ignore health 'hiccups' because they don't feel urgent.

Pay attention to how you feel throughout the day. Are you tired all the time? Do you have trouble sleeping? These could be signs that something needs adjustment.

Don't overwhelm yourself with drastic changes. Start small and celebrate each victory, no matter how small. And make it fun; taking care of your health shouldn't feel like a punishment. Find ways to make it enjoyable.

Your health is your most valuable asset. Every day is a chance to improve your health, one small step at a time. Listen to your body, find what works for you, and enjoy the journey to a healthier you.

Fill Your Cup First

A beautiful, sturdy cup that holds all the love, kindness, and energy you have to give. This cup is you. It's full to the brim when you're feeling good, recovered, and ready to face the world. But what happens when you constantly pour from that cup without ever filling it back up?

You don't have to be everything to everyone.

Many of us, especially those with big hearts, fall into the trap of neglecting ourselves. We take care of family, friends, work, and everything on our plate, forgetting that we're human, too, with needs and desires. We can't pour from an empty cup. When we're depleted, stressed, and running on fumes, our ability to care for others suffers.

So, how do you break this cycle? How do you become a giver who also nourishes yourself? The answer is simple, yet sometimes the hardest - self-care.

Self-care is the foundation for a healthy, happy life and a life where you can truly show up for the people you love. On an airplane, they tell you to put on your oxygen mask first before helping others. It's the same principle. You can't effectively help someone else if you're gasping for air yourself.

Self-care doesn't have to be grand gestures or expensive spa days. It's about the small, daily choices that add up to big results.

We all need downtime to decompress and recharge. This could be getting a good night's sleep, taking a relaxing bath, or simply spending some time doing nothing. Don't feel guilty about prioritising your own recovery time. It's not laziness; it's essential for your well-being.

Make time for activities that bring you joy. Carve out space for things that make your heart sing. It's okay to say no. You don't have to be everything to everyone. Learn to set boundaries at work, in relationships, and with your time. This will allow you to focus on what truly matters and avoid burnout.

Humans are social creatures. Nurture your relationships with loved ones. Spend quality time with friends and family, and join a club or group that aligns with your interests. Strong social connections are very important for happiness and well-being.

Taking a few minutes each day to be present in the moment will work wonders. Try meditation, deep breathing exercises, or focusing on your senses. Mindfulness helps reduce stress, improve focus, and cultivate inner peace.

There will be days when self-care falls by the wayside. Don't beat yourself up about it. Just pick yourself up and try again tomorrow.

As you prioritise self-care, you'll be surprised at how much more you have to give to the world. By taking care of yourself, you're not just doing yourself a favour; you're making yourself a better friend, family member, partner, or colleague. You'll have more patience, more energy, and more love to give to the people who matter most. So, fill your cup, dear friend.

Pick up that mug, fill it with something good, and take a sip. You deserve it!

You Deserve It

You shower kindness on everyone around you but forget about yourself? You're like a sunshine maker, spreading warmth everywhere! But guess what? You deserve that sunshine, too. Remember, a happy you make a happy world around you. So go on, fill your own cup with love and care. You deserve it!

Love Thy Neighbour, But Know Thyself

You heard the phrase, "Love thy neighbour as thyself." It's a beautiful sentiment, encouraging you to care for others as much as you care for yourself. But what happens when this advice is taken too literally? When you prioritise the needs of others above your own, does it lead to a more fulfilling life? Or does it create a toxic cycle of self-sacrifice?

You can't give what you don't have.

If someone tells you to forget about your loved ones and focus solely on yourself, most people would likely react with shock and disbelief. How could anyone suggest such a selfish and heartless thing? We're social creatures, wired to form bonds and connections. Our families and friends are a vital part of our identity and well-being. To abandon them would be unthinkable.

Now, flip the question around and ask someone to put their loved ones before themselves. This time, the response is more likely to be positive. Most people would agree that it's important to be selfless and to prioritise the needs of others.

So, why is it so difficult for us to choose ourselves over others? Why do we feel guilty or selfish when we prioritise our own needs? The answer lies in the way we are raised and the values instilled in us by society. From childhood, many of us are taught to be kind and selfless. We learn to share our toys, help others, and place the needs of our loved ones above our own. This behaviour is praised and rewarded. We feel proud when we do things for others, and we receive positive feedback for our selflessness. We're taught that putting others first is a sign of love and compassion. But the truth is, you can't give what you don't have.

If you are happy and healthy, you create an environment of happiness and health around you.

What You Give Yourself, You Invite Others to Give You

Value yourself;
be valued.

How you treat yourself sets the tone for how others will treat you. When you respect yourself, others notice and respect you, too. If you show love and care towards yourself, people around you will respond with love and care. The energy you give to yourself attracts people who respond in kind. Being kind to yourself shows others how you expect to be treated. When you value yourself, others learn to value you, too.

I'll take care of myself for you, and you take care of yourself for me.

'"I'll take care of me for you, you take care of you for me" – Jim Rohn.' Family first! No time for myself gotta take care of everyone else! I hear this all the time. Putting yourself last is not the noble path, *"Taking care of me strengthens me to take care of you."* This simple shift made all the difference in my life.

Taking care of me
strengthens me to take
care of you.

Your greatest contribution to your family is your own development. When you invest in yourself, your whole family thrives. Self-sacrifice, where you constantly put yourself last, leads to resentment. But self-development and self-investment, where you nourish your own well-being earn respect from yourself and those around you.

Self-love is the source of everything that is.

Commit to self-improvement. It's not selfish, it's heroic! By becoming a stronger, happier you, you become a stronger, happier foundation for your whole family. And that's a story with a happy ending for everyone!

Question?

Who do you love the most in the world? Who is the most important person in your life?

Think of 4 people you love the most. Write their names in order, starting with the person you love the most.

Do not turn the page until you have written those names.

1.

2.

3.

4.

Now, if your name isn't at the very top, or even worse, if it isn't on that list, you have some serious thinking to do.

There is only one choice you make that matters, and that's not to lose yourself in others.

Why wouldn't you love yourself? Why aren't you the most important person in your life? Your happiness and well-being are the most important things. You can only love others if you love yourself first. Yet, you haven't even included yourself on the list.

This is all about you. Everything in life starts with you. If you don't love yourself, you can't truly love others. You can't show real love, kindness, and understanding to anyone, even to those you say you love the most.

But if you did write your name at the top of the list, my friend, then you're on the right track to a happy and healthy life.

First Find It, Then Share It

Happiness is found where you seek it. Start with yourself.

Happiness is a feeling, not a thing you can buy or hold. You can't feel it for others or share it until you first find it in yourself. Trying to light a dark room with a candle that isn't lit—it doesn't work. If you don't feel happiness in your own heart, it's hard to make someone else happy. Once you find that happiness inside, it becomes easier to spread it to those around you, but first, you must find your own happiness.

"Love yourself first, and everything else falls into line. You really have to love yourself to get anything done in this world." — *Lucille Ball*

"No one can make you feel bad if you feel good about yourself." - Michelle Obama

Every Problem is a Good Problem

A businessman and a friend owned a small coffee shop that was frequented by the locals. His coffee was the talk of the town, and people loved coming in for a cup of his special brew.

> *When we fail to see a problem as a problem, we hinder our ability to find a solution.*

One day, a new coffee chain opened up across the street from his shop. The chain offered a wide variety of flavours and a cosy atmosphere that attracted many of my friend's customers. At first, he didn't see this as a problem. He thought his loyal customers would never leave him for a new place.

As days turned into weeks, he noticed a decline in his sales. Fewer people were coming to his shop, and he struggled to make ends meet. Instead of seeing this as a problem, he brushed it off as a temporary setback. He believed that his quality coffee would win back his customers eventually.

However, as months went by, the situation worsened. His shop was on the brink of closing down. It was then that he realised that he had failed to see the problem staring him in the face. His refusal to acknowledge the competition and adapt to the changing market had led to his downfall.

In the end, his coffee shop had to close its doors, leaving him devastated and filled with regret. He wished he had seen the problem earlier and taken action to find a solution.

That day, my friend's story taught me an important lesson – every problem is a good problem. When we fail to see a problem as a problem, we hinder our ability to find a solution. Problems are not roadblocks; they are opportunities for growth and improvement.

People don't see health issues as a problem; that's why they don't care about them.

In our lives, we often encounter challenges that we choose to ignore or downplay. Whether it's in business, relationships, or personal health, turning a blind eye to problems only makes them grow bigger and more difficult to overcome.

Many people neglect their health because they don't see it as a problem. They ignore warning signs, postpone check-ups, and indulge in unhealthy habits, believing that everything will be fine.

The reality is that health issues left unaddressed always escalate and lead to serious consequences. By neglecting your health, you are setting yourself up for potential harm and hardships in the future.

Every problem, no matter how small it may seem, requires attention and action. By acknowledging a problem for what it is, you empower yourself to seek out solutions and make positive changes in your life.

Just as my friend's failure to address the competition led to the downfall of his coffee shop, ignoring problems in any aspect of life has negative repercussions.

People don't see health issues as a problem; that's why they don't care about them. But by shifting your perspective and viewing problems as valuable challenges, you will pave the way for a brighter and more successful future.

Pennies to Panic

Let me tell you another real-life story that happened at my workplace. A colleague of mine fell victim to a scam and lost $300. Here's how it happened.

Every problem, no matter how small it may seem, is a good problem. It's an opportunity to make things right.

One morning, while on his way to work, he received a message on his phone saying that $0.10 had been deducted from his account. Thinking it was such a tiny amount, he paid no attention and ignored it. Not long after, he received another notification about a $2 transaction. He brushed this off, too, considering it to be just another small amount.

But then, his phone buzzed again. This time, with a message stating, "You made a transaction of $300 on your card." That was when he realised something was seriously wrong. He immediately called his bank and took action to secure his account.

Luckily, he acted quickly when $300 was taken. Imagine if he had waited and $3,000 or more disappeared before he noticed. It could have been much worse!

Lesson: Ignoring a small problem leads to a much bigger one down the line. Every problem, no matter how small it may seem, is a good problem because it's an opportunity to make things right. Don't overlook those small signs that are warning you of a bigger issue.

Every Hiccup is a Hurrah

Life, bless its messy glory, throws a whole lot our way. Sometimes, it's sunshine and lollipops, other times, it's flat tyres and overflowing laundry baskets. But the secret most successful folks have learned is that every single thing, good, bad, and in-between, is actually a good problem.

If your car sputtered to a stop (the flat tyre problem), you wouldn't learn how to change a tyre, right? You might be late for work, sure, but you also gain a valuable skill. Problems, big or small, are like road signs. They point out that something needs fixing, a chance to learn and grow.

Of course, some problems feel overwhelming. A job loss, a health concern – these are serious challenges. Even in these moments, there's room for a positive perspective. A job loss is an opportunity to explore a new career path. A health concern is a wake-up call to take better care of yourself. Every problem holds the potential for growth if you allow yourself to see it.

Don't ignore problems or pretend they don't exist. Acknowledge them and then ask yourself, "What's the problem trying to tell me? What can I learn from this? And what new possibilities does this open up?"

Problems are inevitable. They're part of the adventure of life. But by seeing them as good problems, you unlock a whole new way of dealing with them. You become a problem-solver, not a problem-avoider.

Think of it like building a muscle. The more you use a muscle, the stronger it gets. The same goes for your problem-solving skills. The more problems you tackle, the better you become at finding solutions. And that's a skill that will serve you well your whole life.

Next time you face a problem, big or small, take a deep breath and give yourself a little mental high 5. It's a good problem! It's an opportunity to learn, to grow, and to become the best version of yourself.

The Burn That Builds

We've all been there. You step into the gym and stare down the mountain of weights, treadmills, and machines. A knot forms in your stomach. Maybe it's the memory of the last workout's soreness, the fear of pushing yourself too hard, or the unknown. Whatever it is, one thing's for sure: working out is painful.

With each lift, with each push and pull, something amazing happens.

A little bit of pain is a good thing. It's a sign you're pushing yourself, breaking down barriers, and ultimately building something stronger. It's a truth that applies far beyond the gym walls. Discomfort, challenge, and even a little pain are the catalysts for the most significant changes in our lives.

Let's take that workout pain literally for a moment. When you lift weights, you're creating tiny tears in your muscle fibres. It doesn't sound pleasant, does it? But your body reacts by repairing those tears and, in the process, building stronger, more resilient muscles.

The soreness you feel is just a temporary side effect of this incredible growth process.

When you lift a weight for the first time, it feels heavy and awkward. Your muscles strain, and your form will be off. But with each lift, with each push and pull, something amazing happens. Your body adapts. It gets stronger and more efficient. The weight that once felt like a burden becomes manageable. The pain lessens, replaced by a feeling of accomplishment.

This principle extends beyond the physical. When you learn a new skill, it feels awkward and challenging at first. Your brain, like your muscles, is being pushed outside its comfort zone. You'll make mistakes, feel frustrated, and even doubt your ability to learn. But with persistence, those initial stumbles pave the way for mastery.

The Transformation Beyond the Gym

The next time you feel the burn during a workout, it's not just about building muscle. It's a metaphor for life. It's the ache of progress, the discomfort of growth, the pain that paves the way for a stronger, more capable you. The greatest transformations begin with a little bit of pain.

Why does a little pain matter so much? Because it's a signal that change is happening.

This journey of pushing past boundaries isn't always easy. There will be days when the pain feels overwhelming, and you'll want to give up. But keep in mind that the strongest, most resilient people aren't those who avoid pain but those who use it to become their best selves. So put your shoes on, step into the gym of life, and embrace the burn. It will be painful, but it's a beautiful sign that you're changing, growing, and becoming the best version of yourself.

So, why does a little pain matter so much? Because it's a signal that change is happening. Change is uncomfortable, but the payoff is worth it.

A Lifelong Journey to Health

For as long as I can remember, living well has been a priority. Back in the early 2000s, I decided to give my health a major overhaul. It's been over 20 years, and I'm still on this adventure! I've experimented with different diets and exercise routines, all in the name of feeling my best.

Things were quite different back then. The internet wasn't what it is today. Finding health information meant flipping through magazines and books. With limited knowledge, figuring out how to take care of myself was a challenge.

Fast forward to today, and things are a whole lot easier. The internet and social media are overflowing with health advice. But with so much out there, it's easy to get overloaded and confused. Even science has made leaps and bounds, and what we thought was healthy years ago isn't true anymore.

So, what's the secret to staying healthy? The perfect diet or workout plan? Over the years, I've tried many, some with success. But sticking with them long-term proved difficult. They were complicated and left me drained. I realised I needed something simpler, something I could maintain for the long haul.

Maybe you think I'm after shortcuts because I want things easy, but who doesn't, right? Getting healthy isn't always easy, but there are ways to make it smoother if we look for them.

My passion for health has always driven me to learn and discover new ways to improve. Being healthy isn't about the easy way out; it's about finding simple ways to reach your goals. It's about enjoying the journey, challenges and all.

This book is a culmination of my 20-year health odyssey. It's a story of lessons learned, progress made, and the realisation that health is a lifelong journey requiring constant learning and adjustments. It's not about perfection but about balance and well-being.

Through trial and error, I've discovered that simplicity is key. Making healthy choices easy and sustainable is the key to long-term success. I've explored various approaches, always looking for ways to streamline my routine.

The abundance of information can be overwhelming. Sorting through conflicting advice can be a struggle. I've learned to find reliable sources and focus on what truly matters for my health.

Science on health and food keeps changing. Staying up-to-date and open to new information is important so you can make informed choices about your health.

Despite the challenges, I'm committed to my health journey. It's not just about physical fitness; it's about mental and emotional well-being, too. Finding balance in all aspects of life is key to living a healthy and fulfilling life.

The road to success is bumpy. But if we find ways to make the journey easier, we can overcome obstacles. The right tools and mindset help us navigate challenges and get closer to our goals.

I've discovered 4 simple yet powerful rules that have transformed my health over the past 20 years. Later in this book, I'm going to share these simple rules with you.

Success is Health, Health is Success

In my years of chasing dreams and helping others achieve theirs, I've come to realise that true success isn't just about the fancy cars or the trophies on the shelf. It's about feeling your best, both inside and out.

Success is health; health is success.

Think about it: if you're not feeling well, how can you truly give your all? How can you chase those big goals with all your might? That's why taking care of yourself – your body, mind, and spirit – is the real secret to winning at life.

True health means taking care of your emotions, your stress levels, and even your sense of purpose. It's about feeling good in your own skin and having the energy to chase your dreams.

Your health is your greatest treasure. Invest in it, nurture it, and watch how it becomes the fuel that propels you towards all that you desire. Remember, *success is health, health is success.*

Happiness is Health, Health is Happiness

You can't have one without the other. It's hard to separate happiness from health because they feed into each other. Happiness lights up our minds, and when our minds are bright, our bodies respond positively. We cannot chase one without catching the other.

When you are happy, you are healthy; when you are healthy, you are happy. When you are successful, you are happy; when you are happy, you are successful. When you are healthy, you are successful; when you are successful, you are healthy.

When you're happy, you try new things, work hard, and strive to achieve more because you believe in yourself. Success, in turn, brings happiness. You feel proud of your achievements, and this pride boosts your spirit. When you are strong in body and mind, no task seems too big. You can focus better and bounce back from setbacks.

Health, happiness, and success support each other. Without one, the others can't exist. When you take care of your health, happiness follows. When you're happy, your efforts lead to success. And as you succeed, you realise the value of both health and happiness.

A happy heart fuels a healthy body, a strong body helps you achieve goals, and reaching goals boosts happiness. They are companions in this journey of life.

Coffee Club

Have you ever felt the frustration of wanting to exercise but being too busy or tired to make it happen? That's exactly what happened to my friend. He desperately wanted to hit the gym daily, but work and fatigue kept getting in the way.

To do something consistently, you need a routine. To establish a routine, you need motivation. And to find motivation, you need a strong reason, a 'why' behind your actions.

One day, he confided in me about his struggle. He said, "Shah, I just can't seem to find the time and energy to exercise after work. Mornings seem like the best option, but I just can't get myself out of bed to go to the gym."

I listened carefully, then asked him a simple question: "What's the first thing you enjoy doing in the morning?"

"Coffee," he replied without hesitation. "I love my morning cup of joy."

I suggested, "Buddy, what if we started meeting at the gym every morning at 6 am, not to work out, but just to have coffee together?"

He looked surprised. "Just for coffee? But wouldn't that be a waste of a trip to the gym?"

"Trust me," I assured him, "it's part of the plan."

The next morning, he arrived right on time. We sat together, enjoying our coffee and watching people work out. We chatted for about an hour, catching up and having a good laugh. As he got ready to leave, he couldn't help but ask again, "Shah, I still don't understand. Why are we here just for coffee?"

I smiled and said, "See you tomorrow for coffee, buddy."

This routine continued for 3 weeks. Every morning at 6 am, we met at the gym, had our coffee, and talked. After the third week, something amazing happened. My friend walked in, not in his usual clothes, but in gym attire.

"Shah," he announced with a grin, "I woke up before my alarm this morning feeling energised and happy. I knew we were meeting for coffee, but today, I just felt like working out, too."

That's when I explained the power of 'habit'. The reason he couldn't get up for exercise in the past was because he lacked the motivation or a strong enough reason. The thought of working out itself felt overwhelming.

By establishing the coffee routine, we created a habit. Getting up early and going to the gym became a natural part of his day, just like having his morning coffee. Now that the habit was formed, he was ready for the next step – actually working out.

To do something consistently, you need a routine. To establish a routine, you need motivation. And to find motivation, you need a strong reason, a 'why' behind your actions.

So, what's your 'why' when it comes to fitness? Do you want more energy throughout the day? Improve your sleep? Build strength and endurance? Find your reason for wanting to exercise, whether it's better health, weight loss, or simply feeling good. That reason will spark the motivation to create a routine, and soon, getting to work out will feel as natural as that first cup of coffee. Once you discover your reason, the motivation to build a healthy habit will follow.

Building a new habit takes time and effort. But with a clear reason, a positive approach, and a bit of creativity, you can overcome the hurdles and achieve your fitness goals. Now, go out there and find your 'coffee club' moment.

You Don't Need a Therapist, You Need a PT

I've seen many people making good money seem to have it all, but they're just not happy. They're overweight, tired all the time, feeling down and depressed.

> *A healthy body is a strong foundation for a happy mind.*

Sure, some people say mental health is the most important thing. And that's true; our minds are powerful. But our bodies and minds are actually a team. Just like a soccer team plays better when everyone works together, we function better when we take care of both our physical and mental health.

However, I believe a healthy body is a strong foundation for a happy mind.

Taking care of your body first (physical health) can actually be a big boost for your mind (mental health).

You eat healthy foods and exercise regularly. You feel strong energised, and your clothes fit great. This feels good, right? It boosts your confidence. You even start looking forward to trying new things. That's your mental health getting a lift because of your physical health.

Taking care of your body has a ripple effect. When you eat nutritious food, your brain gets the fuel it needs to work at its best. You feel more focused, energetic, and ready to tackle challenges. Exercise is like a natural mood booster. It releases endorphins, these chemicals in your brain that make you feel happy and relaxed. Plus, when you're physically fit, you tend to have more energy throughout the day, which will help you fight off feelings of tiredness and low mood.

Taking care of your physical health builds confidence. When you see yourself getting stronger, fitter, and healthier, it gives you a sense of accomplishment. You start to believe in yourself more, and that is a powerful weapon against depression and other mental health struggles.

Now, this doesn't mean mental health isn't important. There are times when someone might need professional help for serious mental health issues. But for many of us, taking care of our physical health is a powerful first step towards feeling better overall.

So, instead of just talking about your problems, focus on your body. Because, my friend, you might not need a therapist; you might need a PT.

There's no Shame

The only shame is in letting confusion hold you back.

Curiosity is a powerful tool. Dive into a new subject, wrestle with it, and see how far you can get on your own. There's a thrill in the 'aha!' moment when a concept clicks. But sometimes, even the bravest explorers need a guide. Don't be afraid to raise your hand. Asking for help isn't a surrender; it's a chance to learn from someone who's already walked the path. A good teacher can clear the fog and point you in the right direction. The only shame is in letting confusion hold you back.

Knowledge is not Motivation

"Knowledge is power." It's true; knowing things gives you options. But knowing something isn't the same as doing it. Just like a map won't get you to a treasure without taking a step, knowledge alone won't make you fit or happy. That's where motivation comes in, like the fire in your engine.

You know all the fancy names of the machines, but that won't make you lift weights. You need that drive, that spark that makes you want to sweat and push yourself. It could be the desire to feel stronger, look better, or have more energy to chase your kids around. That's motivation – the fuel that gets you moving.

Knowledge is great, but without the motivation to act, it gathers dust in the corner of your mind like a forgotten book.

Motivation is not Knowledge

You've seen them – the super motivated gym-goers, there every day, pumping iron with pure determination. It's inspiring! But just because someone's bursting with motivation doesn't mean they're a fitness pro. Motivation is like a powerful engine in your car, but without the right knowledge, you will end up lost, stalled, or even wrecked.

You are super pumped to lift weights every day. Pushing yourself hard, but if you don't know which exercises target specific muscles or how to use proper form, all that effort isn't doing you much good. You'll be working the wrong muscles, not challenging yourself enough, or worse, risking injury. It's like putting all your energy into driving the wrong way on the highway – you'll eventually get somewhere, but it won't be where you intended.

Learn From the Climbers, Not the Fellow Hikers

My mum, bless her heart, got her driver's licence. But let me tell you, driving wasn't exactly her strong suit. She could pass the test, sure, but on the road? It was a whole other story. The point is that having a fancy certificate doesn't always mean that you are good at it.

Imagine taking driving lessons from someone who's never driven themselves. They might know the rules from a book, but can they handle a nervous driver on a busy street? It's the same with anything you want to learn in life.

You want to climb a mountain. You want to reach the peak, the very top. Who would you ask for help? A person who's already climbed it, right?

This applies to everything, from money matters to getting in shape. If you need a financial adviser, don't just pick someone with a fancy degree. Ask if they've built their own wealth! The same goes for a personal trainer. Sure, they have a certificate, but did they use those techniques to get themselves in top shape?

A piece of paper can only tell you so much. Don't get me wrong, education and credentials are important. But real-world experience is a whole other level. Look for the people who have walked the path you want to walk. They've faced challenges, made mistakes, and learned from them. They can tell you what worked for them and, even more importantly, what didn't. That's the kind of teacher you want in your corner.

Of course, there's always something to learn from everyone. But when it comes to reaching your goals, find people who have climbed the mountain themselves. They'll be the ones to show you the way, not just someone who's looking at the peak with you from the bottom.

Sneaky Monsters

There is a saying, "You are what you eat." It makes sense; the food we put in our bodies fuels us and keeps us healthy. But what if I told you there's another factor that plays a bigger role in our overall health and well-being than the food itself - the sneaky monsters - your emotions.

Sure, sugary treats and endless bags of chips won't help your waistline. But sometimes, our feelings trick us into eating more than our bodies actually need.

Sneaky monsters that make us crave comfort foods – things high in sugar, fat, and calories. They give a short-term mood boost, but they don't solve the problem. Feeling down? We use food like a hug, but it doesn't last. This emotional eating becomes a cycle; stress and sadness lead to food, then guilt, then more stress and sadness. You end up feeling worse after.

SAD B****

Sometimes, there are unexpected guests at the dinner table who can influence your weight more than the food itself. I call them the "SAD B****": (S) Stress that makes you crave comfort food, (A) Anxiety filling you with worry, (D) Depression weighing you down, and (B) Boredom is a B****

(S)

Stress - Tough day at work, traffic jams, and a never-ending to-do list. Exhausted and overwhelmed, what sounds appealing? A light salad? Probably not. Stress triggers cravings for comfort foods — things high in sugar, fat, and calories. They give a temporary mood boost, but they don't solve the underlying stress. In fact, they leave you feeling sluggish and guilty later.

(A)

Anxiety - This monster makes you feel restless and on edge. Feeling anxious is like having a swarm of butterflies fluttering in your stomach. It's a jittery, nervous feeling that is hard to shake. And guess what? It leads to mindless snacking. You reach for food to calm yourself down, even if you're not truly hungry. It's a way to try to control the anxious feelings, but it rarely works.

(D)

Depression - Depression affects eating habits in different ways. Some people lose their appetite when they're feeling down, while others turn to food for comfort. Unfortunately, comfort foods lack the nutrients your body needs, leaving you feeling even worse in the long run.

(B****)

Boredom - We've all been there – stuck at home with nothing to do, scrolling through social media and feeling utterly bored. Boredom is a major trigger for mindless eating. You find yourself reaching for snacks, not because you're hungry, but simply because you're looking for something to do.

So, what can you do? Learn to listen to your body's true hunger cues, not just your emotions. When a craving hits, ask yourself, "Am I truly hungry, or am I just trying to eat away my feelings?" There are healthier ways to deal with emotions. Take a walk, listen to music, talk to a friend, or work on a creative project.

Food is your ally, not your enemy! By developing a healthy relationship with food and finding healthy ways to manage your emotions, you'll take control at the dinner table. You'll not only look better, but you'll feel better, too.

The Past is a Picture

People always show me pictures. Photos of themselves years ago, toned and strong, radiating health. They tell stories of regular workouts, clean eating, and feeling fantastic. I nod along, impressed by their past dedication.

You can choose to linger on the 'good old days' or pick yourself up and start creating a brighter future. But then comes the question: "So, what happened?"

Suddenly, the smiles fade. "Life happened," they sigh. Excuses start rolling in: "Work got crazy," "Family keeps me busy," or "Just can't find the time anymore."

I get it. Life throws punches, that's for sure. Jobs get demanding; families require attention. But these excuses sound like ways to explain away a past glory rather than owning up to the present. See, the past is like a photograph. It's a frozen moment in time. Great, you were fit then, but what about now?

The real power lies in the present. You can choose to linger on the 'good old days' or pick yourself up and start creating a brighter future.

It's not easy. We all crave that extra hour in the day, but everyone has the same 24 hours. It's not about having time; it's about making time. Because trust me, a healthier you have more energy to tackle life's challenges. It's never too late to create a more vibrant picture of yourself.

I once read an old Buddhist story: Two monks were walking by a river on their way home. They heard a young woman in a wedding dress crying near the river. She was sad because she had to cross the river for her wedding, but she was afraid of ruining her dress.

Monks had a rule forbidding them from touching women. But one monk felt sorry for her. He decided to help, picked her up, and carried her across the river. The woman was grateful and thanked him. The monk went back to join his friend.

The other monk was very upset. "Why did you do that?" he asked. "We aren't supposed to touch women!"

The first monk stayed quiet, while the second one kept complaining all the way to their home. He enjoyed the sunshine and birds instead. Back at the monastery, he slept but was woken up by his angry friend.

"Why did you carry the woman?" his friend asked. "Someone else could have helped. You did wrong."

The sleepy monk asked, "Which woman?"

"The one you carried across the river!" said his friend.

The monk laughed and said, "I only carried her across the river. You carried her all the way back here."

Lesson: Let go of the past; leave it at the river.

A monk once said: "Imagine being bitten by a snake, and instead of focusing on healing from the poison, you chase the snake to understand why it bit you and to prove that you didn't deserve it."

Reprogramme Your Mind

Your mind is like an iceberg. The tip sticking out is your conscious mind, the part that makes decisions and plans. But below the surface lies a giant hidden world – the subconscious mind. This powerful force controls your habits, emotions, and how you see the world.

It's like a computer program running in the background. Always working, even when you sleep. It stores all your beliefs, memories, and past experiences. This programme is super strong and influences everything you do, from your mood to your habits. By feeding your subconscious positive thoughts and goals, you can reprogram it for success. It's like replacing old, buggy software with a shiny new update.

Affirmations like "I am strong" and "I am capable" will trick the subconscious into believing them. Imagining yourself achieving your goals can make you feel more confident and motivated. The more vivid the image, the more the subconscious believes it's possible.

This subconscious mind is your biggest cheerleader and worst enemy. Feed it positive thoughts about your goals, and it will secretly guide you towards success. Feed it with negativity, and it will destroy you.

You must learn not to let your thoughts control you; you must gain control of your thoughts.

Thoughts, like trains, constantly arrive. You choose which ones to board. Don't jump on the negativity express! Instead, focus on the positive platform. Look for thoughts of courage, confidence, and joy. It takes practice, but with each empowering thought you choose, you become the conductor of your own happiness. So, take charge, and let only the best trains take you on your incredible journey. You are the conductor, not the passenger.

Shift Your Focus, Shift Your Stress

You are ready for a workout. Your muscles groan, your lungs burn – it feels stressful, right? Yet, we often enjoy it! Why? Because we see the positive outcome – a stronger, healthier us. It's all about perception.

The same goes for life's challenges. When you choose to view life through a positive lens, the weight of stress lightens. Again, it's all about perception. When you see challenges as threats, stress takes hold. But when you see them as stepping stones to growth and achievement, a sense of excitement takes over.

Stress Less, See More

Life throws a lot our way, some big and scary, some small and annoying. The event itself doesn't cause stress; it's how we see it, our perception.

Spilling your coffee. One person gets upset and feels their day is ruined. Another laughs it off, grabs a napkin, and sees it as a chance for a quick break to freshen up. It's all about perception. The same situation can feel completely different depending on how you choose to see it.

It's not about pretending problems don't exist but about finding the good side, even if it's small.

Your perception acts like a filter. A negative filter can turn a flat tyre into a ruined day, while a positive one sees it as an excuse to explore a new walking route. It's not about pretending problems don't exist but about finding the good side, even if it's small. The rain clouds mean a cosy night with a book. You can't control everything that happens, but you can control how you react, and that can make all the difference between a stressful day and a happy one.

You Have to Fail First to Succeed

We get scared sometimes. Fear of messing up, being rejected, or getting laughed at can stop us cold. But failing isn't the worst thing. It's actually a chance to learn and grow stronger.

Failing is a normal part of getting good at anything.

Most people see failing as something bad, something to avoid at all costs. Failing is a normal part of getting good at anything.

One of the best things failing teaches us is how to keep going. When you fail, you pick yourself up, try again, and learn from your mistakes. Without ever tasting something bitter, how would you know how sweet success really is?

Failing teaches us humility. It reminds us that we're not perfect and that everyone makes mistakes. Realising you made a mistake pushes you to work harder, to never give up, and to always try to be better.

When you fail, things get tough. It tests you and shows you how strong you really are. Failing makes you think outside the box. You have to come up with new ideas to reach your goals.

It will show you your weaknesses. This doesn't sound good, but it's actually a good thing! Now you know what you need to work on to improve yourself.

Failing reminds you that success doesn't come easy. You have to work hard for it, fight for it, and give it your all. It shows you the effort it takes to reach your dreams.

Failing lights a fire under you. You want to prove to everyone (and yourself!) that you can do great things. This drive pushes you to achieve amazing things you never thought possible.

So next time you fail, don't see it as the end. See it as a stepping stone on your way to success. Learn from it, grow from it, and use it to jump even higher. Remember, you have to fail first to succeed.

Perfect Isn't Real

Those moments when we want everything to be perfect. We think that if it's perfect, everyone will like it, and it will be just right. We wait for the perfect moment or the perfect conditions to start something, and in waiting, we do nothing at all.

Perfection makes us imperfect. Don't aim for perfection; it's a disaster.

As far back as I can remember, whenever I tried to do something perfectly, I ended up failing or never even started. How many times have you not tried something just because you thought it couldn't be perfect? Many people suffer from this idea that unless something is perfect, it's not worth trying.

But here's the truth: the idea of things being 'perfect' is a lie. Perfect doesn't exist. We chase this ghost called 'perfect', thinking it will make us happy or successful. It doesn't.

What is perfect anyway? Can anyone define it? The answer is no because it's different for everyone, and that makes it an impossible standard.

Practice doesn't make perfect; practice makes permanent.

Real people and real lives are messy, funny, and sometimes a bit broken. That's what makes life interesting and fun. As you stop chasing perfect, you start chasing real life. Don't aim for perfection; it's a disaster. Chase progress, not perfection.

Ever wondered how a story from your past reads differently now? Time to find out!

Once upon a time, in a land of rolling hills and juicy grapes, lived a cunning fox. Whispers of the most delicious grapes imaginable reached his ears, and the fox couldn't resist the chance to taste them. He set off on a quest, his mouth watering with anticipation.

The things we want most are the hardest to reach.

After a long journey, the fox found the vine, heavy with plump, purple grapes. They hung just out of reach, and the fox's eyes sparkled with desire. He leapt and jumped, determined to snag a handful, but no matter how hard he tried, they remained frustratingly high. Disappointment gnawed at him.

He wouldn't give up! The fox tried again and again, but each attempt ended the same way. As his efforts failed, his frustration turned into something sour: envy. He glared at the grapes, muttering, "These grapes are way too high up anyway. They can't be that good." He started making excuses, blaming the vine's height for his struggles. "It's not my fault they're so far away," he grumbled, shifting the blame.

The sun began to set, and the fox's excuses grew wilder. "The branch is too slippery!" he complained. Then, "The wind keeps shaking the vine; that's why I can't grab them!" He desperately searched for anything to blame but himself. His pride was hurt. He couldn't admit defeat.

His frustration boiled over. He even criticised the grapes themselves. "They're probably sour grapes anyway," he scoffed, trying to convince himself they weren't worth the effort. But deep down, he knew they were delicious, and his inability to reach them only made him feel worse.

Night fell, and the fox slunk away from the vineyard, his stomach empty and his heart heavy. His pride was wounded, and his excuses only made him bitter. The next day, he returned, hoping the grapes would magically be lower. But alas, they were just as out of reach, and the fox's excuses became even more creative.

"I tripped on a rock, that's why I couldn't jump higher," he muttered, clinging to anything but the truth. Each excuse was a shield against his own shortcomings. Days turned into weeks, and the fox's excuses became a habit.

Excuses and blame only hold us back, while humility and perseverance lead to sweet success.

One day, a wise old owl hooted at the fox. "My friend," it said, "the grapes aren't to blame, nor is the vine. It's your pride and refusal to see your limits that keep you from enjoying their sweetness." The fox, surprised by the owl's wisdom, stopped to listen.

The owl's words hit him hard. He realised he'd been so busy making excuses and blaming others that he hadn't faced his own limitations. With a newfound humility, he thanked the owl and went back to the vine. This time, instead of excuses, he accepted the vine's height and focused on a solution.

Thinking hard, the fox gathered leaves and made a makeshift ladder. Carefully and determined, he climbed it and finally reached the grapes. As he savoured their sweetness, a sense of accomplishment washed over him, far sweeter than any bitterness he'd felt before.

Excuses and blame only hold us back, while humility and perseverance lead to sweet success. The only thing preventing you from reaching your goals is your own lack of trying. Sometimes, we get so fixated on achieving things in a particular way that we miss other opportunities that could be easier and just as rewarding. It's okay to adjust your approach and accept help when needed.

It's easy to blame external factors, but true success comes from accepting your limitations, trying new things, and never giving up on what we desire. Don't let excuses turn sweet dreams into sour grapes.

Excuses

Oh, how we love them. They feel soft and cosy, like fluffy clouds. We use them a lot, hoping they'll hide our mistakes from others. Excuses are so common, they seem normal. But do they help us grow?

> *Fear and self-doubt are just illusory monsters, not the fire-breathing dragons you make them out to be.*

Those seemingly harmless justifications you offer for your shortcomings and failures have a much more profound impact on your life than you realise. They become like a bad friend who always holds you back. They hug your dreams too tightly so they can't grow. When you use excuses, you choose to stay safe and avoid trying new things. This keeps you stuck in the same place, never reaching your full potential.

Excuses are like protective shields you create to shield yourself from the terrifying monsters of fear and self-doubt. You convince yourself that it's better to stay in your cosy bubble of excuses rather than face the unknown. But fear and self-doubt are just illusionary monsters, not the fire-breathing dragons you make them out to be. Once you understand that, you will tear down your excuse walls and face your fears.

Excuses are familiar to us all. We use them to explain why we didn't do something or to make our choices sound good. However, what remains unspoken is the underlying truth about excuses – they are a choice. They are not merely explanations for your inaction or lack of progress; they are conscious choices you make to prioritise comfort over growth and easy over hard.

Chain Link

They start out as little reasons why you haven't done something, but soon, they turn into a big chain that holds you back from your dreams. Each excuse is a link in that chain, and the more links you add, the harder it is to break free.

> *Each excuse is a link in that chain, and the more links you add, the harder it is to break free.*

Want to start your own business? 'No time' or 'No money' sounds like good reasons to wait. But as time passes, more excuses pile up: "What if I fail?" or "I don't know enough." The dream fades away.

"I'll start exercising next week," but weeks turn into months with excuses like, "I'm out of shape" or "I can't stick to a plan." You remain unhappy with your health.

The scary part is that excuses become a habit. The more you make them, the more you believe you can't change or overcome challenges.

The first step to breaking free is to recognise your excuses. Listen to yourself and catch them when they pop up. Once you see them for what they are - limitations you put on yourself - you will break the chain.

Instead of "I don't have time," say, "I'll work out for 15 minutes every day." Think you're out of shape to exercise? Start small. Take a walk. Focus on learning and growing.

Breaking the excuse trap is about seeing things differently. Excuses aren't facts; they're just your way of looking at things. You can change your perspective.

Excuses We Make

"I don't have enough time." This is common. We all juggle busy lives, but even small changes make a big difference. A 10-minute walk is better than no walk at all!

"It's not the right time." There's no perfect moment! Start today, even with something simple. You'll be glad you did.

"I don't have the resources." Healthy living doesn't need fancy gyms or expensive foods.

"It's too hard." Start small and gradually increase difficulty. Celebrate your progress, no matter how small!

"It's just not meant for me." It's about finding what works for you. Experiment and find activities you enjoy.

"Other people will judge me." Forget about what others might think. Most people are busy with their own lives and won't judge you for trying to be yourself. Focus on yourself and your goals – that's what truly matters.

"I'm too old for it." There is no 'too' when it comes to dreams. You're not too old, too young, too tired, or too anything else. You're exactly who and what you need to be.

"I'm waiting for the perfect opportunity." The perfect opportunity is today! Don't wait for some magical moment to start.

"I've already failed before, so why bother?" Everyone makes mistakes! Learn from them and get back on track. Every day is a fresh start.

"I'll start tomorrow." Why wait? Start today, even with something small. Taking that first step is the most important one.

"The best time to plant a tree was 20 years ago. The second-best time is now." – Chinese Proverb

Excuses = Responsibilities - Effort + Blame

Excuses = Fear + Avoidance − Accountability

Excuses = Procrastination + Denial - Ownership

Where There's a Will, There's a Workout

I have an inspiring story for you. There was a tall, well-built guy I saw at the gym. He had impressive muscles and seemed very dedicated. But he only appeared on weekends.

Dreams are worth chasing, even if the road isn't easy.

One day, I couldn't help but ask him why. I said, "Buddy, I only see you on weekends. Don't you work out on other days?" His answer surprised me. He smiled and said, "Yes, I only work out on weekends because I love it. But I can't afford a gym membership."

He explained that his friend had a membership with a special benefit. This friend could bring one guest for free on weekends. So, he used this opportunity to go to the gym every weekend. I was amazed by his dedication and creativity.

Your health is an investment, not an expense.

He found a way to pursue his passion for fitness. He didn't let a lack of money stop him. Obstacles are only challenges waiting for solutions. Dreams are worth chasing, even if the road isn't easy.

When I Lost All of My Excuses, I Found My Results

When you stop making excuses, you'll realise one thing: you are unstoppable.

For a long time, I had reasons why things wouldn't work. I wasn't ready, the time wasn't right, or something else always got in the way. But then, I stopped making excuses. I just started doing the thing I wanted, even when it felt scary. And guess what? I actually got things done. It turns out excuses were holding me back. Now, I see my efforts turn into results, and it feels amazing.

Why Can't You Just Say, 'I Lost'?

I had a coworker, let's call him Tom. Tom had a peculiar way of talking about games. Whenever you asked him who won, if he was the winner, he'd excitedly shout, "I won!" His face would light up with joy. It was clear that victory made him feel proud and happy.

People don't want to accept their mistakes and failures. It feels too painful, too shameful.

But if someone asked him who won when he lost, his answer would always be, "Oh, the score was 100 to 95," or some other score. No signs of disappointment, just numbers, as if the numbers could somehow soften the blow of defeat. He never mentioned who actually won if it wasn't him.

I noticed this pattern and started to wonder why he did that. Why does he act this way? Why couldn't he just say, "I lost"? I couldn't quite figure it out completely. But mostly, people do this for the following reasons.

Couldn't Admit Defeat:

Admitting you lost is hard. It makes people feel sad and weak. People find it really tough to say, "I lost." They think losing means they are not good enough. So, they try to hide it by not saying it directly.

Couldn't Accept Someone Else Winning:

In any game, only one person or team can win. When someone else wins, it means you didn't. For people, accepting this is difficult. They want to be the winner all the time. Seeing someone else win makes them feel upset.

> *Life is like a big game, and to win it, we need to learn from our losses.*

Everyone loses sometimes. It's a part of life. When you don't accept your losses, you don't learn from them.

You miss the chance to become better. On the other hand, no one wants to be around someone who can't be happy for others. Being able to cheer for other people's success shows you are kind and supportive.

In life, it's important to accept both winning and losing. Winning feels great, but losing teaches you valuable lessons. It helps you understand what you need to do to get better. When you learn from your losses, you truly win in life.

Tom's way of handling games was a small thing, but it made me think a lot. It showed that how we act can tell us a lot about how we deal with life. Life is like a big game, and to win it, we need to learn from our losses.

Everything in life is intertwined with our mental, physical, and emotional well-being. Each part of our life, like our choices and behaviour, affects how we feel and live.

Let me explain. When you can't admit defeat, it affects your mental health by making you feel anxious and stressed. You worry about how others see you and your self-worth. This mental stress impacts your physical health. Emotionally, avoiding the truth leads to feelings of disappointment and sadness, lowering your confidence and making you hesitant to try again.

When you struggle to accept others' success, you compare yourself to them. This makes you feel jealous and inadequate, negatively affecting your mental well-being. The jealousy and comparison increase stress, putting your body in 'fight or flight' mode, which again leads to physical problems down the line. Emotionally, being unable to celebrate others' achievements results in feelings of isolation and loneliness and damages your relationships, causing further emotional disconnect.

Tired & Trapped

We see it – the shiny new cars, the sprawling houses, the endless stream of 'stuff'. We are all caught up in chasing the latest luxury.

But what good is a dream home if you're too tired to enjoy it? Or a fancy car if you can't even get behind the wheel because you're not feeling well? It's a sad reality, but most people prioritise possessions over their own well-being.

Health isn't a luxury; it's a necessity. It's the gift that keeps on giving, allowing you to live life to the fullest and truly appreciate everything else you have.

Beyond What Eyes See

The old woman sat by the window, watching the world. Cars hummed, children shrieked, leaves danced. But her gaze held a curious distance. Her granddaughter asked, "Grandma, what are you looking at?"

Sometimes, the most real things are the ones we can only feel.

The woman smiled, a touch sad. "The world, child. But it's not quite what you see. It's a symphony of whispers, a dance of unseen threads. We walk through it, but most never see the real story."

The child tilted her head, confused. "But Grandma, it's right there!"

The woman chuckled. "Yes, love, it's right there. But sometimes, the most real things are the ones we can only feel."

The Gift of Time

Old and wise, looking back on your life. What matters most in that moment? Money? A fancy car? A bigger house? No. All we truly crave at the end is more time. Time to laugh with loved ones. Time to chase dreams. Time to simply exist.

Don't wait until it's too late. Seize the day! Every minute is a gift. Don't let it slip through your fingers. Money can't buy more minutes; fancy cars can't rewind the clock. The only treasure you can't get back is time itself. Invest your time in what truly matters. Because, in the end, that's all you'll have left to treasure. When the time runs out, all that will be left are the memories you make along the way. Make your time count.

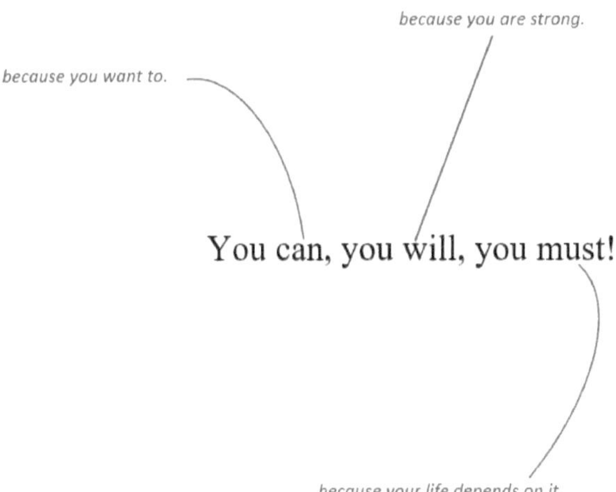
because you are strong.
because you want to.
You can, you will, you must!
because your life depends on it.

2

Myths & Mistakes

Have you ever heard someone say that cracking your knuckles gives you arthritis or that sugar turns kids into bouncing beans? The world of health is full of strange ideas, many of them simply not true. These are called health myths, and they can be really confusing.

Just because someone says something with confidence doesn't mean they're right.

A lot of us hear these myths from friends, family, or even on the news and social media. We think, 'Well, they must know something', and take it as fact. But the biggest mistake you can make is to believe everything you hear without checking it out yourself.

Just because someone says something with confidence doesn't mean they're right. Do your research, ask questions, and find out the truth. Your health is important, and you deserve to make informed decisions.

Myth #1

Skipping Meals

Eat less, move more. When it comes to weight loss and healthy living, it sounds simple enough, right? But for many, the 'eat less' part gets twisted into something unhealthy – skipping meals altogether. It seems like a logical leap – less food equals less weight, right? Well, hold on a minute! While this approach seems quick and easy, it's actually a recipe for disaster when it comes to healthy weight loss and overall well-being.

Skipping meals will cause the scale to dip, but what you're losing might not be what you think.

Food is the fuel, and your metabolism is the engine that burns that fuel to keep you going. When you don't eat enough, your body feels threatened, like it's entering 'starvation mode'. In this mode, your metabolism actually slows down to conserve energy. This means you burn fewer calories overall, making weight loss even harder.

Skipping meals will cause the scales to dip, but what you're losing might not be what you think. Instead of burning fat, your body starts breaking down muscle for energy. Muscle is metabolically active, meaning it burns calories even during recovery. Losing muscle slows down your metabolism even further, making it even harder to lose weight in the long run.

Your body is incredibly smart. When you deprive yourself of food for long periods, your hunger hormones go into overdrive. This leads to intense cravings and episodes of overeating later on. It's a vicious cycle – you skip meals, your body screams for food, you overeat, and then feel guilty, starting the whole cycle over again.

Food is your body's fuel. When you don't eat enough, you're essentially running on fumes. This leads to fatigue, low energy levels, and difficulty concentrating. Skipping meals reduces your body's ability to function throughout the day.

Think about your health goals beyond just a number on the scale. Aim to feel energised, focused, and strong. After all, it's not about depriving yourself but about nourishing your body for the amazing things it can do. Eat right, eat less, eat when you're hungry and stop when you're comfortably full. Eating is not a problem; overeating is.

Myth #2

The Eight-Glass Myth

Water. It's the very essence of life, a cool refreshment on a hot day, and the foundation for a healthy body. We've all heard the advice: drink 8 glasses of water a day. But is this a golden rule etched in stone or a health myth that needs a refresh? The eight-glass rule is more like a friendly suggestion than a scientific fact.

Water is the king of hydration, but it's not the only player on the team.

Believe it or not, the eight-glasses-a-day advice doesn't have a rock-solid scientific foundation. It likely stems from recommendations made back in the 1940s, suggesting a daily fluid intake of around 2.5 litres (that's about 8.5 glasses). While not entirely off the mark, this advice wasn't based on a specific study of water needs but rather a general estimate.

Another theory suggests the eight-glass rule emerged from early nutritional studies that focused on healthy adults in temperate climates. These studies looked at average fluid intake and did not consider factors like individual differences in activity level, body size, or even climate.

We're all unique! Our bodies function differently, and our water needs vary greatly. Many factors influence how much water you actually need, like activity level, climate, body size, and diet. If you're a couch potato, your water needs will be different from someone who runs marathons. Exercise leads to sweating, which means you need to replenish those lost fluids.

Living in a hot, humid climate naturally makes you sweat more, requiring more water intake. Conversely, colder climates do not necessitate the same level of hydration. Larger bodies generally require more water than smaller ones. If you eat a lot of fruits and vegetables, you're already getting some water content from your food. However, a diet high in processed foods leaves you needing more water for overall hydration.

Instead of rigidly following the eight-glass rule, your best bet is to listen to your body's natural thirst cues. Water is the king of hydration, but it's not the only player on the team.

Water is vital, but it's not the whole picture. Electrolytes are minerals like sodium, potassium, and magnesium that help your body function properly, including muscle and nerve function. When you sweat a lot, you lose electrolytes, too. So, while water replenishes fluids, consider including electrolyte-rich options (watch the sugar content), coconut water, or even a pinch of salt in your water, especially during intense activities.

The eight-glass rule isn't a one-size-fits-all solution. Understand your body's unique needs and listen to its thirst cues to ensure proper hydration. Experiment with different strategies, find what works for you, and enjoy the benefits of being a well-hydrated, healthy you.

Myth #3

Carbs: Friend or Foe?

For many of us, carbohydrates, or 'carbs' for short, have become the enemy on our journey to a healthy weight. You hear stories of people shedding pounds after cutting carbs, and shelves are overflowing with 'low-carb' everything. Carbs aren't inherently bad. In fact, they're a crucial part of a balanced diet.

If you eat more calories than your body burns, you'll gain weight, regardless of when you eat those calories.

Carbs Make You Fat. This is a widespread belief, but it's not true. Carbs themselves aren't the villain in the weight gain story. The real culprit is consuming more calories than your body burns each day.

Calories are the fuel for your body, and you burn them throughout the day for energy. If you pump more fuel (calories) into your body than it burns, the extra fuel gets stored – that's weight gain. Now, the type of fuel you use matters. Some fuels, like sugary drinks, burn quickly and leave you wanting more soon after. Others, like complex carbs, provide sustained energy and keep you feeling fuller for longer.

So, carbs aren't bad. In fact, they're an essential part of a healthy diet. Your bodies break down carbs into glucose, which is the primary fuel for your brain and muscles. Your bodies need carbs to function properly.

Moderation is key. Eating excessive amounts of any food, even healthy carbs, will lead to weight gain. The trick is to choose the right types of carbs and eat them in appropriate portions.

There are 2 main types of carbs: simple and complex. Simple carbs are like the sugary snacks I mentioned earlier. They're quickly digested by the body, causing a spike in blood sugar levels. This quick burst of energy is followed by a crash, leaving you feeling hungry again soon after.

Complex carbs, on the other hand, are the good guys. They're packed with fibre, vitamins and minerals. Unlike their simple counterparts, complex carbs break down slowly, providing sustained energy and keeping you feeling fuller for longer. This helps you eat less overall, promoting healthy weight management.

Fibre is a magical ingredient in complex carbs. Not only does it keep you feeling satisfied, but it also has other health benefits. Fibre helps with digestion, keeps your blood sugar levels stable, and even lowers your risk of heart disease.

While drastically cutting carbs leads to initial weight loss, it's not sustainable in the long run. Carbs provide your body with energy for exercise and everyday activities. Without them, you'll feel sluggish and struggle to maintain a healthy routine. Additionally, restrictive diets are difficult to stick to, leading to cravings and potential overeating later.

Another myth: 'Don't eat carbs after sunset' for weight loss? This popular belief can leave you confused about what to eat for dinner. There's no magical time limit for enjoying carbs.

The idea behind the 'no carbs after dinner' rule is that our bodies stop burning calories efficiently at night, leading to weight gain if we eat carbs. However, this isn't quite accurate. Your bodies use energy (calories) all the time, even when you're sleeping. While your metabolic rate slows down a bit at night, it's still burning calories to keep you alive and functioning.

If you eat more calories than your body burns, you'll gain weight, regardless of when you eat those calories. Carbs are an essential part of a healthy diet. They provide your body with energy for everything you do, from powering your brain to keeping your muscles working.

Interestingly, complex carbs before bed are actually beneficial for sleep. These carbs promote the production of tryptophan, an amino acid that helps your body produce the sleep hormone melatonin. So, a small snack with complex carbs before bed even helps you drift off to dreamland faster.

If you're still concerned about evening carb intake, try having your larger, carb-rich meal earlier in the day, like at lunch. This gives your body more time to burn off the energy from those carbs before bedtime.

The Bottom Line is that carbs are not the enemy. By choosing complex carbs, prioritising fibre, and practising portion control, you can enjoy a healthy, balanced diet that fuels your body and supports your weight loss goals. It's the total calories you consume, not just where those calories come from. Listen to your body, choose healthy options, and enjoy all the delicious foods nature has to offer.

Myth #4

Weight Training Makes Women Look Like Bodybuilders.

My friend, Maya, was staring longingly at a picture in a fitness magazine. "Ugh, I wish I had her toned arms," she sighed, flopping down on the couch.

"Why don't you work out?" I suggested, taking a sip of my tea. Maya's face scrunched up. "Work out? No way! I don't want to get all bulky like those bodybuilders."

I smiled, understanding her fear. This was a common fear I heard, especially from women. "Hold on a sec," I said, putting my tea down. "There's a big misconception about lifting weights. Lifting weights won't make you look like a man."

Maya raised an eyebrow. "Really? But what about all those women with huge muscles?"

"It's not that simple," I explained. "Let's break it down," I said, grabbing a pen and napkin. "First, building massive muscles takes years of dedicated training, a specific diet, and sometimes even special supplements. It's not something that just happens by accident."

I drew a simple circle on the napkin. "Think of your muscles like this. Now, imagine lifting weights makes the circle a little bit bigger." I drew a slightly larger circle next to the first. "That's what happens when you work out. Your muscles get a little stronger, a little more toned."

Maya nodded, following along. "Okay, so a little bigger, not huge."

"'Exactly! Now, those bodybuilders you see? They've pushed their circles way, way out," I drew a huge circle dwarfing the others. "It's an extreme.'"

"But why wouldn't women want to look strong?" Maya asked, tilting her head.

"Strong is great! But there's a difference between strong and bulky. Lifting weights can actually help you look toned and lean, which is what most women are aiming for anyway."

I sketched a curvy figure on the napkin. "See how the lines are smooth? That's what toned muscles look like. They give your body a nice shape and definition."

Maya was starting to look more convinced. "So, lifting weights won't make me look like a man?"

"Nope! Women naturally have much lower levels of testosterone, the hormone that helps build big muscles. It's just basic science."

"Wow, I never knew that," Maya admitted. "So, what would lifting weights actually do for me?"

"Great question!" I said, happy to see her curiosity piqued. Here's the good stuff: lifting weights actually has a tonne of benefits, especially for women.

First, it helps you build lean muscle. Muscle burns more calories than fat, even during recovery. This means your body becomes a more efficient calorie-burning machine, even when you're not actively working out.

Second, stronger muscles support your bones better. This is especially important as you age, as it helps prevent injuries and keeps you feeling strong and independent.

Third, lifting weights improves your posture, which not only looks good but also helps with things like back pain and headaches.

Fourth, it boosts your metabolism. The more muscle you have, the faster your body burns calories. This is a huge help if you're trying to lose weight or maintain a healthy weight.

Fifth, and most importantly, lifting weights makes you feel amazing! It gives you a sense of accomplishment and boosts your confidence. You'll feel stronger, more capable, and ready to take on anything.

"Wow, that sounds pretty awesome," Maya admitted. "But what kind of weights should I even use? And what exercises?"

I smiled. "There's a whole world of weight training out there, but don't worry, it doesn't have to be complicated. Start with bodyweight exercises. As you get stronger, gradually add free weights."

"And the gym isn't the only option, right?" Maya asked.

"Absolutely not!" I said. The key is to find something you enjoy and can stick with.

"I could give it a try," Maya said, a determined look in her eyes. "Just some light weights at home to start?"

"Perfect!" I said, giving her a high 5. "Remember, it's not about getting bulky, it's about getting healthy, strong, and feeling good about yourself. And trust me, you won't regret it!" Maya was excited, and I knew she'd do great.

Don't let the myth of getting bulky hold you back. After all, lifting weights isn't about becoming a bodybuilder; it's about taking control of your health and creating the strongest, healthiest version of yourself. You'll surprise yourself with how strong and capable you are.

Weight Loss

Losing weight can feel like a confusing maze. But shedding pounds boils down to one core principle: managing your calorie intake. Simple, right? Well, simple in theory, perhaps. But, like most worthwhile things in life, it takes a bit of understanding and effort to put it into practice.

When it comes to weight loss, it doesn't matter what you eat; it's how much you eat.

Your body is like a bank. Calories are like money you deposit. If you deposit more than you withdraw, you gain weight, like a growing account balance. To lose weight, you need to flip that scenario. You need to burn more calories than you take in, creating a 'calorie deficit' that makes the body tap into its stored reserves (fat) to fuel itself.

When you use more calories than you take in, your body dips into its stored reserves, causing weight loss. The opposite happens when you take in more calories than you burn; the excess gets stored as fat.

Let's assume you need 2,500 calories a day, and if you only eat 2,000 calories from an ice cream, you will lose weight. Why? Because you're burning 500 more calories than you're putting in. Sure, you can lose weight by eating only ice cream, not the healthiest way to lose weight, but I hope you got the idea. When it comes to weight loss, it doesn't matter what you eat; it's how many calories you eat. It's simple math: burn more calories than you consume, and your weight will follow.

So, how many calories should you aim for? It depends on a few factors: your age, sex, current weight, activity level, and goals. Generally, women tend to require fewer calories than men, and someone who exercises intensely will burn more calories. You don't need to be a math whiz to calculate all that; there are plenty of online calculators and apps that can estimate your daily calorie needs for weight loss.

Now, how do you control this calorie intake? Food! Food is amazing. It fuels our bodies and brings joy to our taste buds. But some foods pack more of a caloric punch than others.

One simple strategy is portion control. Our eyes are bigger than our stomachs. Pay attention to serving sizes. Use smaller plates to avoid piling on extra food.

Not all calories are created equal. A giant bag of chips might have the same number of calories as a salmon salad, but the salad offers a wealth of vitamins, minerals, and fibre that keep you feeling fuller for longer.

The truth is blunt: to lose weight, you need to burn more than you consume. Your withdrawals need to be bigger than your deposits. That's a calorie deficit, plain and simple. That's it. No magic, just basic math.

Understanding the Two Faces of Fat Burning

Burning fat for energy is like using a log to make a fire. When your body needs energy, it uses the fat you eat and the fat stored in your body. Imagine a little worker inside you going to the fat storage room to get some fuel for the body.

Your body doesn't just burn fat to shed weight; it also fuels you with energy.

But burning stored fat is a different story. It's like finding an old treasure chest in the attic. Your body taps into the stored fat when it doesn't get enough energy from the food you eat. It's like a backup plan for your body, saving fat for a rainy day.

When you exercise and go without eating for a while, your body starts burning the stored fat. It's like using up the emergency savings when money is tight. This helps in losing weight and reducing body fat.

So, burning fat for energy is normal and happens all the time to keep you going. It's a natural process that your body undergoes to survive and stay healthy.

Your body doesn't just burn fat to shed weight; it also fuels you with energy. It's like a power-up button that keeps you going throughout the day, powering your every move and thought.

Burn More While You Recover

Many believe that running for miles or hitting the spin bike is the only way to slim down. But that's not quite true! While cardio, like running or swimming, is great for your heart and lungs, it's not the weight loss champion some might think.

The weapon for shedding pounds is actually building muscle.

The weapon for shedding pounds is actually building muscle. When you lift weights, you build muscle. Muscle burns more calories than fat and gives your body a metabolism boost. This means you burn more calories even when you're recovering! So, the more muscle you have, the more calorie-burning machine your body becomes.

Cardio is still important for overall health. But if weight loss is your goal, think about adding some muscle-building exercises to your routine.

Gift From Nature

Muscles make you stronger and help you look younger. You see, muscles have many benefits. They support your body. They help you move. Strong muscles protect your bones and joints. When you have good muscles, everyday tasks become easier.

As we grow older, our muscles naturally get smaller and weaker. This process is called sarcopenia. If you do not work on building muscles, this will make you feel weak and fragile.

One of the big benefits of having strong muscles is that it helps you stay independent as you grow older. For example, it becomes easier to get up from a chair, walk without falling, or carry your groceries. You can do more things on your own without needing help from others. This independence is very important for a happy and fulfilling life.

Muscles are the secret to a long and healthy life. Having strong muscles improves your balance. It helps prevent falls, which are common in older adults.

Muscles make you stronger, healthier, and more independent. Working on building muscles is one of the best things you can do for your future self. Muscles are a gift from nature.

The Age-Defying Duo

Our bodies produce amazing chemicals called hormones. These affect how young we feel and look! One, testosterone, is like a special power for men. It helps keep muscles strong and skin firm, making them look younger. Women have less testosterone, but they have another hero hormone: growth hormone, called GH. This amazing GH helps keep skin plump and bright, giving women a fresh look.

These hormones play a crucial role in keeping muscles strong and skin firm and promoting overall vitality, helping you look and feel younger than your age.

Eating healthily and regular exercise keep your body strong and help it produce more testosterone and growth hormone. There's no magic potion for eternal youth. But by eating well and staying active, you give your body the tools it needs to keep those youthful hormones flowing. So, if you want to keep that youthful look, focus on healthy food and exercise. It's like a natural fountain of youth for both men and women!

Let's Not Go Against It

Many people love to party and stay awake late. They think the night is for fun, laughter, and joy. Cities are bright and alive even after the sun sets. Lights, music, and celebrations are everywhere. It feels like nighttime is full of energy.

But what does nature tell us? Night is dark and silent. This is nature's way of saying it is time to recover, just like how the sun rises and sets, your body has a natural rhythm. When the sun goes down, your body wants to sleep. Sleep helps you heal and get ready for the next day.

During the day, the sun fills the world with light, and the world becomes lively. This is the time for work and activities. The day is for learning, working, and experiencing life. Nature designed it this way for a reason. Your brains work better, and you feel strong and motivated when you follow this pattern.

Staying awake at night confuses your body. It is like trying to swim against a strong current. Listening to nature helps you stay balanced and healthy.

Let the night be a time for peace and recovery. Enjoy the day with all its opportunities. Trust what nature wants for us. The night is a gift for recovery, and the day is a blessing for work. Nature knows best. Let's not go against it.

Shake Things Up a Bit

Stuck in a rut? Like life's on repeat, same days, same routines, same outcomes? Well, there's a reason for that. If you keep doing the exact same things, guess what? You'll keep getting the exact same results.

Doing the same thing and expecting different results, it just won't happen.

If you want to see different results and different experiences, you have to start doing things differently. It is scary at first, stepping outside your comfort zone. But that's where the magic happens. Trying new things, even if they seem small, opens doors you never knew existed.

You always take the same route to work. One day, you decide to try a different street. Maybe it's a little longer, but you discover a cool coffee shop, a hidden park you never knew about. Suddenly, your routine feels a little less routine, and your day a little brighter.

Shake things up a bit, try something new. You'll surprise yourself with the amazing results you create.

Now, of course, if you're perfectly happy with your current results, then keep on keeping on! There's nothing wrong with a good routine as long as it brings you joy.

Same Old Recipe

To truly create something different, you need new rules to guide your actions.

I always tell people, "Change your rules, change your mindset." They nod their heads in agreement, but then they go on to do the same old thing. Imagine trying a new recipe but using the same old ingredients. To truly create something different, you need new rules to guide your actions. Change starts with you. If you want something different, create new rules for yourself. Don't wait for someone else to set the game. Your life changes when YOU change your rules.

Change and Accept

Change is part of life. Many people switch jobs and hobbies because they feel stuck and bored. It's not that they aren't good; they're caught in a loop, repeating actions that don't work. They keep doing the same things over and over, even if it's not working out.

Your life changes when you change your rules.

When you keep doing the same thing again and again without stopping to think, you can't see your mistakes. You start to think that what you're doing is the right way. You can't see the way out. This is a problem because it stops you from learning and growing. You need to be open to change. Only then can you see your mistakes and make things better.

It's not anything else but your own habits and attitudes that are holding you back. You need to try new things and be open to different perspectives. It's not always easy, but it's the only way to achieve your goals. It's okay to make mistakes. Accepting them allows you to move forward.

4 Mistakes

Mistakes are like little bumps in the road of life. They can sometimes make us feel sad and embarrassed, but they are also a big part of learning and growing. Without making mistakes, we wouldn't know how to do things better.

Life without mistakes would be like trying to paint without colours.

When you make a mistake, be kind to yourself. Instead of getting upset, try to understand what went wrong. You didn't pay enough attention, or you didn't know something you should have. Once you know why you made the mistake, learn from it and try to do better next time.

Without mistakes, you would remain stagnant, trapped in a cycle of repetition. Imagine a world without mistakes – a world where everyone is perfect, where there's no room for error. It would be a dull, lifeless place devoid of the excitement and thrill of discovery.

But to truly benefit from your mistakes, you must first acknowledge them. You need to face them without shame or fear. Once you've acknowledged your errors, the next step is to understand their consequences. What impact did your mistake have on yourself and others?

Nobody is perfect. We are all works in progress, constantly evolving through the mistakes we make and the lessons we learn.

Mistake #1

Focusing on Goals, not Purpose

My first day of fitness instructor training started with a question that's stuck with me ever since. Our instructor, a man with kind eyes and a booming voice, looked at our eager faces and asked, "Why are you here?" We all chorused what we thought he wanted to hear: "To become fitness instructors!" He dropped another question: "Why do you want to be fitness instructors?"

Uncover the deeper purpose that drives you, and you'll find the true north star that guides your journey.

Different voices echoed in the room, each sharing their reasons – "I love fitness, I seek a career in the fitness industry, I aim to change my career path." But it was the instructor's next words that left a lasting impression on me. He said something profound: "That's all well and good, but in life, it's not what you do, it's who you are that matters."

What did he mean? Was he saying our passion for fitness wasn't important? He left us with that question mark hovering over our heads, a mystery to solve.

Years later, it finally dawned on me. All those answers, our desire to be instructors, were goals, not a purpose.

Our purpose is the deeper reason behind our goals. It's the 'why' that fuels our 'what'. You love fitness because it makes you feel strong and joyful. Maybe you dream of a career in fitness because you want to inspire others to feel that same way. That's the purpose hiding within your goals.

Do what you love, but be who you are.

Uncover the deeper purpose that drives you, and you'll find the true north star that guides your journey. It's not just about what you do; it's about who you become in the process.

Goals v/s Purpose

To live a happy and healthy life, the first thing everyone should know is the difference between setting a goal in life and living your life with purpose.

Purpose leads you to the right path. With goals, you choose the wrong direction sometimes just to succeed fast.

People feel stuck and unhappy, not because of life's challenges. Everyone faces challenges; it's part of life. They are unhappy because they lack a strong purpose. They think ticking off goals will make them truly happy. No, it's a purpose that fills life with more joy and meaning.

Goals are like tasks. You set them, you achieve them, and you're done.

Unlike goals, purpose is ongoing – it's not a checklist item. Goals are steps you take, but purpose is the path you walk on.

Purpose gives life direction. Living with purpose means aligning your actions, thoughts, and emotions towards something meaningful. Knowing why you're doing what you're doing. That's what living with purpose means.

And another thing about goals and purpose is that with goals alone, you don't necessarily make the right choices. But when you have a purpose in life, you'll always make the right choices for yourself.

For example, losing 10 pounds is your goal, and you set a target you want to achieve in, let's say, 3 months. You focus so hard on hitting that target that you start taking unhealthy shortcuts. You might take drugs; they will help you achieve your goal, but those are not necessarily good for your health. You're driven by the goal, not what's good for you.

Goals are like finish lines, tempting us to stop running once we cross them.

On the other hand, living a healthy life is a purpose in life. Now, your actions change. You'll be more mindful; you'll make better choices. You'll avoid everything that is not good for your health.

Purpose leads you to the right path. With goals, you choose the wrong direction sometimes just to succeed fast.

Shift your focus from goals to purpose. Purpose is the driving force behind your journey. It's the 'why' that fuels your 'what' and 'how'.

Purpose fills life with meaning and gives you a reason to jump out of bed in the morning. It's not the nagging alarm clock but the internal fire ignited by your core desires.

Find your purpose, find what truly matters to you. Trust me, your life will shine with meaning and joy. It will bring happiness from knowing you are part of something bigger. When you live with purpose, it becomes your internal alarm clock. The desire to fulfil your purpose wakes you up in the morning, eager to take on the day.

Don't Make Hobbies

Hobbies are like a gentle breeze, refreshing and light. People enjoy them in their spare moments, much like sipping coffee on a quiet afternoon. But passion is a fiery force that fuels your soul, demanding attention and dedication. It's what you live for, not just what you do.

When you have a hobby, you do it in your free time. But when you have a passion, you make time for it.

When you have a hobby, you work it into your existing schedule. It's a pleasant part of your life, something you can pick up or set down whenever you choose. It's nice, but it doesn't change anything.

Passion transforms you. It wakes you up in the morning and keeps you up at night. Passion doesn't ask for time; it demands it. It challenges you to rearrange your priorities.

All the successful people who excel in their fields have one thing in common: they don't just love what they do; they live for it. Their passion becomes their purpose, guiding them toward their dreams.

When passion leads, each step feels lighter. Challenges become opportunities, and setbacks become lessons.

Hobbies fill your time; passion fills your life.

Your heart is in it, and that makes all the difference. Passion creates a sense of fulfilment and joy that fills your life with meaning.

"I believe every one of us is born with a purpose. No matter who you are, what you do, or how far you think you have to go, you have been tapped by a force greater than yourself to step into your God-given calling." – Oprah Winfrey

"If you can't figure out your purpose, figure out your passion. For your passion will lead you right into your purpose." – T.D. Jakes

Mistake #2

Distracted

I see people working out at the gym, but instead of focusing on their exercise, they're glued to their phones. They finish a set, grab their phone, and start scrolling through social media. They think they're recovering, but they're actually distracting themselves.

When you're working out, you're investing in your health. You're paying the price, so to speak, with sweat and effort.

When you work out, you're not just exercising your body; you're also training your mind. You need to be focused and determined to push yourself to your limits. When you're constantly checking your phone, your mind is elsewhere. You're not giving your workout the attention it deserves.

When you buy something at a store, and you're paying for the item, you don't just pull out your money without looking. You count the bill and make sure you're paying the right amount. You're paying attention to the transaction.

When you're working out, you're investing in your health. You're paying the price, so to speak, with sweat and effort. Don't waste that investment by being distracted.

Focus on your mission. Don't let anyone or anything distract you. This is your time and your mission. It belongs to you and only you. Keep your eyes on the prize and move forward.

Pay attention to how your body feels. Take a moment to appreciate the progress you've made. This will help you stay focused and motivated. Keep your eyes on the prize, not the phone. Your phone can wait. Your health can't.

Mark Zuckerberg didn't just scroll through social media; he put in the effort to create a powerful social media platform. Steve Jobs didn't simply play with phones; he built a leading company that outshone all other phone companies. Cristiano Ronaldo didn't just sit and watch football on TV. He worked hard and became a famous name in football. Arnold Schwarzenegger didn't just watch others exercise. He worked hard to become the greatest bodybuilder ever.

So, ask yourself this: Do you want to be the one watching or the one who is watched and admired by everyone?

Mistake #3

Shame of Being Less Than Others

One of the biggest hurdles people face on their health journey is self-doubt. Many times, people start comparing themselves with others, whether it's about their weight, how fit they are, or what they can do. They look at others and feel like they don't measure up.

Step by step, day by day. You'll get there.

Comparing yourself to others is like comparing apples to oranges. Everyone's journey is unique, with different starting points, goals, and challenges. When you focus on what others have, you lose sight of your own progress and potential.

Instead of comparing yourself to others, you should compete with them. Instead of thinking that others are better than you, you should see it as a challenge to be better than them. Instead of feeling ashamed of yourself, just do what you need to do and feel proud of yourself. Don't hide from others because you're not as good as them. We think of others as better than us.

But we should not give others this power. Instead, use their strength as your motivation.

Your worth is not determined by your fitness level or your appearance. You are valuable, and your journey is unique.

Mistake #4

Health Seems Like a Simple Fun Activity

You've heard the phrase, "Make it fun, so you'll enjoy it." Many people have misunderstood its real meaning. Making something fun doesn't mean you should forget its importance. It's not about fooling around and leaving the core message behind, especially when we are talking about health.

If your health is on the line, so is everything else. You cannot press pause, and you certainly cannot restart.

Health is a serious game. It's not a video game that you play where you have multiple lives and will always get second chances. Health is real life. If your health is on the line, so is everything else. You cannot press pause, and you certainly cannot restart. Yet, some people treat their health as if it's just a casual joke, something easy to cast aside.

Would you laugh it off if you had to deal with a serious illness? Would you roll your eyes if your body couldn't do what you needed it to do just because you weren't paying attention to it? Probably not, right? It's because, deep down, you know that your life depends on your health and well-being. This isn't about being another health fad or just making fancy resolutions. It's about understanding the weight that your well-being holds in your life.

We live in an era where we take things lightly, sticking to the idea that life is just about being carefree and having fun. But if you want to enjoy life to the fullest, keeping your health a priority is non-negotiable. Making healthy choices isn't something you should dread or avoid. It should be a regular part of life, like brushing your teeth. Sure, find enjoyment in what you do, but with the understanding that it holds significance.

Now, let's not confuse taking it seriously with making it boring or dreadful. The choices you make today will shape your future. Every little decision contributes towards making your life and body better.

I'm being completely serious. Your health deserves your respect. It deserves your attention. It deserves your effort. Don't just make it fun. Make it a priority. This isn't just some random thought; it's a fact. Nobody is asking for the impossible. You're given this one body, this one life. Would you risk it all for the sake of fun? I hope not. Because there is no redo button in life.

'It's Never too Late.' Sometimes it is.

"It's never too late!" It's a comforting thought as if there's an endless supply of chances. But is it always true?

Sometimes, there are no do-overs. You only get one shot.

If you miss the bus, there will be another one coming. If you forget your lunch, you can always buy something to eat. But life isn't always like that.

Life isn't a game with retries. Sometimes, that ache in your chest isn't a passing thing. That nagging cough might not disappear on its own. That tiredness that never goes away might be a warning. Don't wait until it's too late. Don't wait until you get sick or injured to realise how precious your health is.

Sometimes, there are no do-overs. You only get one shot. You can't rewind and try again. The choices you make today affect how you feel tomorrow.

Your health is a precious seed. The sooner you plant it, the stronger the tree will grow. Neglect it, and it will never sprout.

Don't wait for a 'next time' that might not come. This is your health, your well-being, your one shot at this amazing life. Make it count. Don't wait for a wake-up call that might never come. Take care of yourself today, listen to your body and what it's telling you. Because with your health, sometimes there are no second chances, only now or never. Choose wisely.

Why Your Fitness Goals Fail

People struggle to reach their fitness goals, and a lot of it comes down to one thing: expectations.

By setting the bar too low, we limit ourselves. We think we don't deserve it. And setting it too high, we feel disappointed when things don't go as planned.

Marshall Goldsmith identified a few reasons why people fail to achieve their fitness goals. Here are the 4 biggest expectations that don't let people achieve their fitness goals.

Time: It takes a lot longer than they expected.

Effort: It's harder than they expected.

Reward, *I refer to as validation*: After they see some improvement, they don't get the response from others that they expected.

Maintain: Reaching your goal is one thing; maintaining it is another. Not expecting that they'll have to stick with it for life, they gradually regress or quit entirely.

Results, Not Just Effort

Always remember your end goal, but don't expect immediate rewards while you're working hard. Just keep putting in the effort. People get discouraged because they develop expectations. They feel their hard work isn't noticed enough. They think about quitting, not because they lack the ability, but because it seems pointless to continue. Remember, your greatness will be seen in the results, not the process. Your dedication, principles, and determination will be reflected in your achievements, not in the effort itself. It's all about the results, not just the hard work.

Your passion will show in **results**, not in your work.

Your perseverance will show in **_results_**, not in your work.

Your resilience will show in *results*, not in your work.

Your drive will show in ***results***, not in your work.

Your vision will show in **results**, not in your work.

Your focus will show in ***results***, not in your work.

Your courage will show in *results*, not in your work.

Your optimism will show in ***results***, not in your work.

Your gratitude will show in *results*, not in your work.

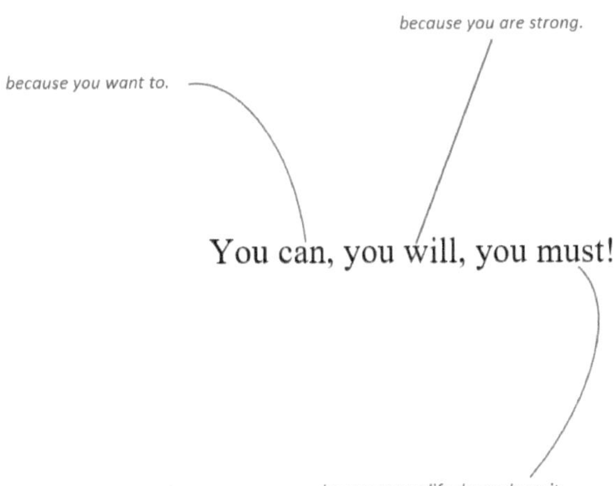
because you are strong.
because you want to.
You can, you will, you must!
because your life depends on it.

3

Rethink the Way You Talk About Health

For too long, the conversation around health has been dominated by illness. We talk about diseases, symptoms, and treatments, creating a narrative of fear and struggle. But what if there was another way? What if we reframed the conversation to focus on wellness, on building resilience and thriving, not just surviving? It's time to rethink how you talk about health, moving towards a more holistic view that considers the whole person – mind, body, and spirit.

Our current health system operates in a reactive mode.

Our current health system operates in a reactive mode. We wait until we get sick, then scramble to find a fix. This can be effective for emergencies, but for long-term health, it's like constantly patching up a leaky roof. A more proactive approach focuses on wellness – building the foundation for good health. It's about creating habits that nurture your body and mind, making you more resilient to illness.

We used to think of the mind and body as separate entities. But they have a deep connection between them. Stress, for example, manifests as physical symptoms like headaches or stomach aches. Similarly, chronic pain leads to anxiety and depression.

Your health is not solely in the hands of doctors and medications. You have immense power to influence your own well-being through the choices you make every day.

The way we talk about health shapes how we think about it.

Health is not created in a vacuum. It's heavily influenced by the social and economic conditions in which we live. Factors like access to healthy food, safe neighbourhoods, quality education, and social support all play a significant role in determining health outcomes. A person living in poverty with limited access to nutritious food and healthcare will likely have poorer health than someone with greater resources. This is why promoting social justice and creating a more equitable society is crucial for improving overall health.

The way you talk about health shapes how you think about it. Instead of focusing on illness and disease, use language that empowers and motivates. Talk about building resilience, cultivating well-being, and thriving in life. This positive approach makes health feel more achievable and creates a sense of agency over your well-being.

Sometimes, despite your best efforts, you get sick. It's important to move away from blaming yourself or feeling like a failure. There will be setbacks and challenges – that's part of life. Practice self-compassion, be kind to yourself when things aren't going smoothly, and focus on getting back on track.

There's no one-size-fits-all approach to health. What works for your best friend might not work for you. Listen to your body and find what makes you feel your best. Maybe you thrive on high-intensity workouts, or a gentle walk in nature is more your style. Perhaps meditation helps you manage stress, or spending time with loved ones is your key to relaxation. Create a health plan that fits your unique needs and preferences.

Your sense of spirit, your connection to something larger than yourself, plays a vital role in overall well-being. Having a sense of purpose, feeling connected to a community, and engaging in activities that bring meaning to life contribute immensely to your health. Whether it's spending time in nature, volunteering, practising a religion, or pursuing a creative passion, nurture your spirit and find what gives your life a sense of purpose.

Rethinking the way you talk about health shifts your entire perspective.

The Game of Life

Life is a game, a grand adventure filled with twists, turns, and unexpected challenges. We all want to win, to achieve our goals and reach for success, but what does winning even mean? Is it always about coming in first, achieving the highest score, or crushing the competition? And what happens when you lose? Does it mean you're a failure? Does it mean the game is over? Not at all. In fact, a crucial part of playing well involves understanding that winning and losing are part of the journey.

When winning becomes the sole objective, it leads to a narrow perspective.

From a young age, we're conditioned to focus on winning. We get gold stars for good grades, trophies for athletic achievements, and high-fives for being 'the best'. This competitive spirit has its place, pushing us to strive for excellence and reach our full potential. However, when winning becomes the sole objective, it leads to a narrow perspective. You overlook valuable lessons learned from losing, become discouraged by setbacks, and experience significant anxiety about not achieving the 'top spot'.

A seesaw. You are on one side, your goals and aspirations on the other. When you 'win', the seesaw tips up, placing you closer to your goals. But what about when you 'lose'? The seesaw dips down, but it doesn't break. Instead, it creates momentum, propelling you back up for another try.

Similarly, life's experiences, both positive and negative, contribute to your growth. You learn from your mistakes and setbacks, becoming more adaptable and resourceful. You discover hidden strengths and develop valuable coping mechanisms through challenging situations. These lessons, learned through 'losing', shape who you become and equip you for future endeavours.

When you focus solely on winning, the emphasis is on the end result, the trophy at the finish line. A more fulfilling approach emphasises the effort, the dedication, and the journey itself. Did you train hard, give your best shot, and learn something valuable along the way? These are the true measures of success, regardless of the final outcome.

Celebrate the small victories along the way. Each step forward, each obstacle overcome, is a cause for pride. Acknowledge your progress, take time to reflect on your efforts, and appreciate how far you've come. This fosters a sense of self-worth and motivation, independent of external validation through winning.

We all face setbacks, disappointments, and moments when we feel like we've 'lost'. It's during these times that developing a sense of resilience is crucial. Neutrality towards winning and losing helps you accept these challenges, learn from them, and bounce back stronger. You learn to navigate through tough times with a positive attitude and the belief that you can overcome anything.

Life is meant to be enjoyed. When you focus on winning at all costs, the pressure to succeed takes away the joy of playing the game. Approach life with curiosity, enthusiasm, and a willingness to take risks. Explore new experiences and learn from both victories and defeats. That's where you'll find true fulfilment.

When we focus on winning at all costs, the pressure to succeed takes away the joy of playing the game.

The key is understanding that winning and losing are 2 sides of the same coin. They create a necessary balance in the game of life. Victories fuel your motivation and provide a sense of accomplishment. Setbacks, on the other hand, build resilience, teach you humility, and push you to improve.

Each step forward, each obstacle overcome, is a cause of pride.

Life isn't just about reaching the finish line. It's about the experiences, connections, and lessons learned along the way.

Beyond Gym Bags and Salads

We live in a world obsessed with external markers of health. We chase six-pack abs and fill our social media feeds with perfectly posed workout pics. But true health goes beyond the gym bag and the salad bowl. The key to lasting well-being lies not in what you do but in who you are at your core and how you think about yourself and your body.

Well-being lies not in what you do but in who you are at your core and how you think about yourself and your body.

Imagine your health as a magnificent garden. Your actions – exercising, eating healthily, getting enough sleep – are like the visible efforts you put in, watering the plants and pulling weeds. But the foundation of this garden, the invisible force that truly determines its beauty and health, lies beneath the surface. It's the fertile soil, the nurturing sunlight, and the unseen seeds waiting to sprout.

These 'seeds' in the garden of health are your thoughts and beliefs. They shape your approach to health and fitness. Positive thoughts about your body, like "I am strong and capable, my body is a temple," act like healthy seeds. These thoughts inspire you to take care of yourself and make healthy choices.

On the other hand, negative thoughts, like "I'm not good enough" or "I'll never be healthy," are like weeds in the garden. They choke out positive motivation. Feeling constantly defeated about your appearance or fitness level makes you give up before you even begin.

Your beliefs about health and fitness are like the root system of your garden. They are the underlying assumptions you hold about yourself and your ability to be healthy. Did you grow up surrounded by healthy habits, or were you exposed to negative messages about food and exercise? These early experiences shape your beliefs, which in turn influence your actions in the present.

Limiting beliefs, like "I'm genetically predisposed to be overweight" or "I'm just not good at exercise," act like weak roots, hindering your growth. They make you feel powerless to change your health and fitness levels.

However, empowering beliefs, like "I can be healthy at any size" and "I can learn to enjoy exercise," become the strong roots that provide support and stability for lasting change. Believing in yourself and your ability to be healthy, regardless of your starting point, is fundamental to achieving and maintaining well-being.

At the very heart of the health garden lies your core being – your authentic self, your essence. This is the part of you that is untouched by external influences and societal pressures. It's the wellspring of self-compassion, resilience, and the desire to feel good in your own skin.

Connecting with your core being is like nourishing the soil in your garden. It provides the fertile ground from which all else grows. When you accept and appreciate your body for what it can do, rather than focusing on what it 'should' look like, you tap into a source of inner strength and motivation.

By focusing on your thoughts, beliefs, and core being, you empower yourself to take charge of your health. You become the gardener.

Trends Won't Make You Healthy

Have you ever scrolled through social media and felt a pang of envy? A friend's picture-perfect smoothie bowl, someone else's ripped abs after trying the latest workout craze? It's easy to get caught up in the highlight reel of other people's lives, feeling like you're missing out on the secret to happiness and health. But chasing trends is a recipe for disappointment.

Focusing on what everyone else is doing steals our focus from what truly matters.

We're bombarded with messages about what we should look like, what we should eat, and what exercises we should do. New 'superfoods' pop up every week, promising eternal youth and workout challenges flood our feeds, guaranteeing a beach body in just 30 days. The problem is these trends are fleeting fads, not sustainable solutions for a healthy life.

Focusing on what everyone else is doing steals your focus from what truly matters – your own body and needs. We all have different preferences, fitness levels, and health backgrounds. What works for one person might not work for you, and constantly comparing yourself leads to frustration and discouragement.

Trends paint an unrealistic picture of health. Those magazine cover bodies are the result of genetics, extreme exercise routines, and even photo editing. Obsessing over achieving that image leads to unhealthy eating habits, injuries from pushing yourself too hard, and a distorted view of what health truly looks like.

Trends are all about the quick fix. They promise instant results, but real health and well-being are about long-term commitment and building sustainable habits. Fad diets and intense workouts give you temporary results, but they're hard to maintain and leave you feeling yo-yo-ing between extremes.

So, what should you do instead? You are the expert on your own body. Pay attention to how different foods make you feel, how much sleep you need, and what types of exercise you enjoy. There's no one-size-fits-all approach.

Every step in the right direction is a victory. Don't get discouraged by setbacks. Building healthy habits takes time and effort. Celebrate small wins. Every step in the right direction is a victory.

Living healthy shouldn't feel like punishment. Find something you genuinely enjoy doing so you'll be more likely to stick with it. Healthy habits shouldn't feel like a temporary challenge. Think about how you can integrate healthy choices into your everyday life. Pack healthy snacks for work, cook meals at home more often, and find ways to be active throughout the day.

Shift your focus from achieving a certain appearance to how healthy choices make you feel. Don't chase fleeting trends – focus on nourishing your body, mind, and spirit for lasting well-being.

True health and happiness come from within. Embrace your own unique journey and let go of the pressure to chase fleeting trends.

Firefighter

For most of our lives, healthcare has been like a fire station. We wait for something to go wrong, a fire to break out in our bodies, and then we rush to the doctor, the firefighter, to put it out. This approach feels a bit reactive, doesn't it? What if, instead of waiting for emergencies, you focused on fire prevention – building a strong, fire-resistant house within yourself? That's the power of wellness. It's about building resilience, a strong foundation for your health. It means taking charge and creating habits that keep you healthy, minimising the chances of getting sick in the first place.

Traditionally, medicine has been like waiting for the fire to start before calling for help. If you get sick, then see a doctor for treatment. But wouldn't it be better to take control and prevent these fires altogether?

A doctor can prescribe medication to fight off the flu, but wouldn't it be better to have a strong immune system that naturally fights it off? Building a strong immune system is a powerful defence against illness.

Many diseases can be prevented or delayed with healthy habits. It's like building firewalls within your body, making it harder for illness to take hold.

When you focus on wellness, you take control of your health. You're not passively waiting for something bad to happen – you're actively creating good health. It's like learning fire safety tips and taking precautions to minimise the risk of a fire starting in your own home.

A focus on wellness goes beyond the physical. It includes mental and emotional well-being, too. Feeling good overall leads to a more fulfilling life, like living in a safe and secure home with peace of mind.

Doctors can offer personalised advice on healthy habits based on your individual needs. They can be your expert consultants, helping you find the best ways to keep your body running smoothly. But the real power is in preventing illness in the first place. Doctors are there, but focusing on wellness is your secret weapon for a strong and healthy you.

Feel Good, Not Just Look Good

We know the importance of healthy food, enough sleep, and regular exercise. But there's another powerful ingredient that gets overlooked, and that is the energy you surround yourself with. Just like the food you eat nourishes your body, the emotional energy you're exposed to has a profound impact on your health and well-being. Move beyond just 'looking good' and focus on 'feeling good'.

The way you talk to yourself matters.

Imagine yourself walking into a room. One room is filled with laughter and lively conversation. People are smiling, and there's a sense of excitement in the air. Now, picture another room. It's quiet, almost tense. People seem withdrawn, and their faces are etched with worry. Which room would you feel more energised and happier in? The answer is clear. Positive energy is contagious. Just like a smile can light up a room, negativity drains the life out of it. We, as humans, are incredibly good at picking up on the emotional cues of those around us. A friend's frown can make you feel concerned, while a colleague's enthusiasm can motivate you.

Science behind it: our brains have mirror neurons, which fire when we observe the actions or emotions of others. When someone is stressed, your mirror neurons pick up on those vibes, and your body starts to react similarly, increasing your stress hormones. On the other hand, positive energy triggers the release of feel-good chemicals like dopamine and oxytocin, which boost your mood and overall well-being.

Be mindful of how you feel after interacting with them. Surround yourself with people who lift you up, make you laugh, and inspire you to be your best self. And don't feel obligated to take on someone else's negativity. If someone is constantly draining your energy, politely excuse yourself - set boundaries.

True health and happiness are about so much more than just looking good.

The way you talk to yourself matters. Replace negative self-criticism with supportive and encouraging thoughts. You are your own best cheerleader. Find activities that make you feel happy and alive.

Helping those in need is a great way to shift your focus away from your own problems and create positive energy. Volunteer your time, donate to a cause you care about, or do something kind for someone else.

In today's world, we focus on looking good on the outside. But true well-being comes from feeling good on the inside. By surrounding yourself with positive energy, you create a foundation for a healthy, happy, and fulfilling life.

So, the next time you're thinking about your health, don't just think about your physical body. Think about your energy, too. Make a conscious effort to surround yourself with positive people and create a positive environment.

After all, true health and happiness are about so much more than just looking good; it's about feeling good from the inside out.

Healthy Habits

Healthy habits aren't just about carrots and crunches. They include your thoughts, actions, and behaviours. When you think positively, it becomes a healthy habit. Being kind and understanding to others is a healthy habit. The way you deal with stress and handle challenges are all parts of living a healthy life. It's about making good choices every day.

The Race Isn't Over

You haven't reached game over. This is just a little halftime slump. The score might not look good right now, but you still have the power to turn this game around.

This game – your game – is far from over. You are in control.

Those excuses are like whispers from the comfort zone, that lazy place where nothing changes. They're comfortable, sure, but they're also suffocating. You deserve to feel strong, to move with ease, to wake up each morning feeling like you can tackle anything.

Look, I get it. Time feels like a precious commodity these days. But instead of dreading the gym, why not start with a walk around the block? Thirty minutes.

That's all it takes to get your blood pumping and your mind clear.

You are never too late or old to start again. You might not win sprinting contests anymore, but there's a whole world of fitness out there waiting to be explored.

Every step you take, every push-up you complete, every healthy choice you make is a victory. You're not just fighting the scale; you're fighting for a better version of yourself. You're proving to yourself and everyone around you that you haven't given up and that the fire still burns brightly inside you.

Don't wait for a magic Monday or a perfect time to begin. Start today. Even the smallest step forward is a step out of the comfort zone. Get out there and show the world what you can do. You are stronger than you think. You are capable of more than you believe. This game - your game - is far from over. You are in control.

It won't be easy, but the rewards are worth every step. So, get up, dust off those forgotten weights, lace up your shoes, and take the first step. Because the game may have gotten a little tougher, but it's definitely not over yet.

Sunrise Sweat v/s Paycheck Chase

I see people raise eyebrows, even chuckle sometimes, at those who rise with the sun to exercise. But that same morning, when those same folks drag themselves out of bed for work to chase that paycheck, suddenly, everyone's cheering them on – "Such a hard worker!" It's strange, isn't it? We treat money like the holy grail, more important than our own health.

> *If you're healthy, you can chase after all the money you desire.*

If you're healthy, you can chase after all the money you desire. But if you're stuck battling health woes, that money loses its shine. It can't buy you back the energy you once had or the joy of moving your body with ease.

Taking care of yourself is the real investment. It's the one that pays off every single day.

Your Health is Harder to Earn Than Your Paycheck

If I ask you a question: what's tougher, earning a good living or living a healthy life? Making a buck or living healthily? Most folks would likely say making money. It's a common belief, this idea that financial success is a never-ending uphill battle. See, that's the thing:

when something feels like a massive struggle, guess what we humans tend to do? We dodge it. It's baked into our nature to avoid discomfort.

If making money truly were the harder task, wouldn't our mornings look a lot different? We wouldn't see millions of people dragging themselves out of bed, gulping down coffee, and scrambling to get to work. We wouldn't have rush hour traffic jams with everyone racing to the office. But how many of those same people do you see waking up before dawn to hit the gym or packing healthy lunches the night before? Not quite as many, right?

That's exactly why living a healthy life takes the top spot for difficulty. It forces you to confront challenges head-on, to break away from comfortable routines, and to make choices that do not always feel good in the moment.

Money is a powerful motivator. We need it to survive, to buy a roof over our heads, food on the table, and all those things that make life comfortable. So, even though it is tough, the reward for earning money is clear.

Living healthily, however, offers a different kind of reward. It's not always immediate gratification, like the joy of a new purchase. It's more like a slow burn. You won't feel the difference right away, but over time, you will have more energy, feel stronger, and avoid health problems down the road. It's a long-term investment in yourself, which can be harder to stick to in the moment.

It's like saving money. You wouldn't expect to become a millionaire overnight, would you? You start small, put away a few bucks each week, and then watch it grow over time. It's the same with health. Small, consistent changes lead to big results, and that's something we can all achieve.

The next time you feel like giving up on that healthy habit, remember it's not about immediate results, it's about building a better you, one small step at a time. And that, my friend, is a reward worth fighting for.

Living healthily is the toughest challenge, but it's the one with the most valuable payoff – a longer, happier, and more fulfilling life.

Millions Mean Nothing if You Can't Move

You win the lottery! Millions in the bank, a world of possibilities. But what if you're ill, too tired to enjoy a trip around the world? True happiness relies on physical well-being, not financial.

Being physically fit is the first step towards being financially fit. Your health is the foundation of everything you do. If you're struggling with extra weight, feeling down, or constantly battling illness, even a mountain of money loses its shine.

Being physically fit is the first step towards being financially fit. If you feel heavy, sad, and unwell, no amount of money in the bank can make you feel better. Your health becomes the most important thing.

All the money in the world cannot buy you good health. Your body is your priceless possession, and taking care of it should be your top priority. When you are physically fit, you can conquer any obstacle that comes your way. So, before thinking about wealth, focus on your health.

When you're physically fit, you feel strong and energetic, sleep better, think sharper, and have the stamina to tackle whatever life throws your way. Now, that big paycheck? It becomes a tool to support your healthy lifestyle and fuel your ambitions. So, while money is important, prioritise your physical well-being. Taking care of yourself today is the best investment you can make for a brighter, healthier, and wealthier future.

Your body is like a precious treasure that needs care and attention. A healthy body is a wealthy asset that money cannot buy. Your well-being is your ultimate wealth, so cherish it like gold.

True Currency of Happiness

They say you can't buy happiness with money. I totally agree with that. Money doesn't bring happiness, but good health does. It lets you enjoy all the good things in life, the things that truly make you happy. When you're feeling strong and full of energy, it's easier to enjoy life's simple pleasures. When you're healthy, you have the energy to do the things you love. You can spend time with loved ones or chase your dreams. Money can't buy that sunshine feeling.

Compassion, not cash, brings contentment.

If money guaranteed joy, we wouldn't hear about celebrities and rich people ending their own lives. Robin Williams, known for making everyone laugh, suffered deeply inside. Despite his success and wealth, he lost his battle with depression. Anthony Bourdain, a famous chef and traveller, explored the world and tasted its finest flavours but still felt empty. Adolf Merckle, who had a net worth of around $9 billion, took his own life. Kate Spade couldn't escape her own sadness. Happiness is found in love, laughter, and caring for ourselves. True happiness is crafted from meaningful connections, fulfilling experiences, and inner peace, not from the dollars in our bank accounts.

Money is not the key to happiness, but good health is. It lets you live your life to the fullest, and that's something money just can't buy.

Free to Breathe, Strong to Choose

You can be poor, with a roof over your head that leaks a little and a dinner table that wobbles but still feel richer than a king. How? By calling the shots on your own life.

Money lines pockets, but it doesn't fill hearts. True wealth isn't just about the numbers in your bank account. It's about the freedom to breathe and the power to choose. You can be poor, with a roof over your head that leaks a little and a dinner table that wobbles but still feel richer than a king. How? By calling the shots on your own life. It's the security of knowing you can fix the leak, tighten the table, and create a life you love. It's the joy of free time spent with loved ones, the thrill of learning a new skill, and the satisfaction of a job well done, even if the pay is small. True wealth whispers, "You may not have much, but you have everything you need to build a life of meaning." It's the quiet hum of purpose that sets your soul alight, money or not.

4 Fundamental 'Fs'

"Wealth is not authored by material possessions, money, or 'stuff,' but by what I call the 3 fundamental 'F's'.

1. Family (relationships)

2. Fitness (health)

3. Freedom (choice)

Within this wealth, trinity is where you will find true wealth and, yes, happiness.

Wealth is strong-spirited familial relationships with people. Not just your family but with people, your community, your God, and your friends. At the end of the iconic movie, It's A Wonderful Life, we're given the final lesson: 'Remember, no man is a failure who has friends'. This reflects on the importance of sharing your life with friends, family, and loved ones. Wealth is making a difference. Wealth is community and impacting the lives of others. Wealth cannot be experienced alone in a vacuum.

Believe me, the richest moments of my life occurred when I was surrounded by a family of friends and loved ones.

Second, wealth is fitness: health, vibrancy, passion, and boundless energy. If you don't have health, you lack wealth. Ask any terminally ill person what they value. Ask any cancer survivor how they suddenly feel reborn and happiness is displaced from 'stuff' to people and experiences. There is no price on health and vibrancy.

And finally, wealth is freedom and choice: freedom to live how you want to live, what, when, and where. Freedom from bosses, alarm clocks, and the pressures of money. Freedom to passionately pursue dreams. Freedom to raise your children as you see fit. And freedom from the drudgery of doing things you hate. Freedom is the liberty to live your life as you please." - Demarco, M.J.

4th F (Fascination)

Your body is amazing. It does so much. You walk, talk, think, and feel with it. Every beat of your heart, every breath you take, is a small miracle. To be fascinated by your body means to be amazed by it. You should be amazed because it is so wonderful and complex. It's like looking at a magic show every day.

When you are fascinated, you care more. You look for answers. This helps you make good choices about your health. You feel eager to try new things. Your mind is busy and happy.

Fascination is like a fire that keeps you warm and eager. So, be fascinated by your body. Explore, learn, and love the amazing body you live in.

4 Feel Good Rituals

Life can be a whirlwind. You rush from one thing to the next, and before you know it, the day is gone. In the midst of all this busyness, it's easy to forget the little things that bring joy and meaning to your life. 4 habits that will help you feel good every day.

Sit Under the Sun for 10 Minutes in the Morning

Getting some sunlight in the morning is a great start to your day. Sunlight helps your body make vitamin D, which is good for your bones and immune system. It lifts your mood and makes you feel warm and happy. The sunlight gives you energy and helps you wake up. Try to find a safe spot outside, a garden or balcony, where you can enjoy the sun. Just 10 minutes is enough. You can sip your coffee, listen to the birds, or watch the clouds. This little time makes a big difference.

Tidy Up, Lighten Up

Waking up to a fresh start every morning. The air feels lighter, and your mind is calm. Decluttering your space is a great way to feel more relaxed and focused. Decluttering your space is like cleaning out your mind. When your surroundings are organised, your thoughts become clear.

A clean area helps your mind feel clear.

Pick one corner of your room or a single drawer. Open it and take a moment to see what's there. You'll find things you forgot existed!

With less clutter around you, you find room to dream, to think, and to grow. You begin to see life's possibilities with more clarity and hope.

A tidy space means fewer distractions. It gives you a sense of control and peace. You'll notice that with less clutter, you find it easier to focus on tasks and relax in your personal time.

This simple habit of organising and tidying will truly transform how you feel every single day. Make your surroundings lighter and your heart happier.

Read a Book

Reading is a wonderful way to relax your mind and expand your knowledge. It takes you to different worlds and lets you meet new characters. Choose a book that interests you, whether it's a mystery, a romance, or a self-help book. Reading helps you escape from every day worries. It improves your focus. Spend some quiet time each day with a book. You can read in the morning, during lunch, or before bed. Even just a few pages are enjoyable and beneficial.

Heartfelt Connections

Connecting with loved ones is the heart's balm in a busy world. Sharing laughter and stories with friends and family makes you feel loved and cherished. These moments remind you of your worth and importance. Whether it's a call, text, or a coffee meet-up, these connections offer comfort and joy. When you spend time with people who care about you, stress melts away. You feel understood and appreciated. Make this a daily habit. It's a small act with big returns.

The Most Amazing Place You'll Ever Be

There's one place I wouldn't want to leave - my own body. Your body is amazing. It's like a whole world, full of wonder and constantly changing. It lets you do so many things: run, jump, hug, dance, sing, taste delicious food, and feel the warmth of the sun. It's strong enough to carry you through your day and clever enough to heal itself from little bumps and scrapes.

There's one place I wouldn't want to leave - my own body.

Your body is your home. It's where you experience everything in life. It carries your thoughts, feelings, and memories. It's the only place you'll ever truly be. So, wouldn't it make sense to take care of this incredible place?

Think about your house. It's a cosy cabin in the woods or a beach house by the sea. It makes you happy, so you want to keep it in good shape, right? You wouldn't let the roof leak or the windows break. You'd fix things when they needed fixing, and you'd clean them regularly to keep them fresh.

Your body works the same way. It needs care to stay strong and healthy. Your body is like a machine that needs fuel to run. The food you eat is like putting gas in the tank. But you wouldn't put junk in a fancy car, would you? Just like a house needs time to settle after a busy day, your body needs to recover. Sleep is when your body repairs itself and gets ready for a new day.

Your body was made to move. Exercise is like playing for your body. It keeps your muscles strong, your bones healthy, and your heart happy. Your body is pretty good at communicating with you. When it's happy and healthy, you feel great.

Your body is your home. It's where you experience everything in life.

Your body is always changing and growing. As you get older, your body will do amazing things like grow taller, develop new skills, and even give you the power to create a whole new life. It's a fantastic journey, and taking care of your body is the best way to make the most of it.

When you feel strong and healthy, you have more energy to do the things you love. You can play with friends, explore new places, and learn new things. Feeling good in your body gives you confidence and makes you feel happy about yourself.

Your body is your best friend, someone you can rely on, someone who's always there for you through thick and thin. It's with you every single moment, helping you experience life.

Respect your body. It's the only one you get.

So, treat your body with respect. Take care of it, listen to it, and give it the love and respect it deserves. Because when you take care of your body, you're taking care of the most amazing place you'll ever be.

The Strongest Pillar

You have grand plans for your house. Each room holds a piece of your heart – a hub for passions, a welcoming space for loved ones, and a sanctuary for your dreams. But what happens if the foundation of this house is weak? Cracks appear, walls wobble, and the whole structure becomes unstable. Just like a house, your health is the foundation on which everything else rests. Without a strong foundation, even the most amazing dreams won't be able to take root.

> *Without a strong foundation, even the most amazing dreams won't be able to take root.*

Think of your health as the sunshine that nourishes a plant. With sunshine, the plant thrives, grows tall, and produces beautiful flowers. When there's no sunshine, the plant withers and struggles to grow.

Have you ever felt tired and sluggish, making it hard to even think about your goals? Good health gives you the energy and stamina to pursue your passions and chase your dreams.

From climbing mountains to dancing the night away, good health allows you to enjoy all the wonderful things life has to offer. You can be active and adventurous and make the most of every moment.

When you're healthy, you have the energy and focus to nurture your relationships with loved ones. You can be present and supportive and create lasting memories together.

As you get older, good health becomes even more important. It allows you to stay independent, take care of yourself, and continue living life on your own terms. Just like a building with a weak foundation can crumble, neglecting your health has serious consequences.

The healthier you are, the more you enjoy life, chase your dreams, and make a difference in the world. It's like building a strong foundation for the amazing life you want to live.

Making your health a priority, you are building the strongest possible foundation for a happy, fulfilling life. A healthy you is a stronger, more confident you, ready to take on the world.

Love, Respect and Accept

These words sound more like something you'd hear about in a relationship advice column or things for greeting cards, but they're actually powerful tools for your health journey.

Loving yourself is listening to your body's whispers, not shouts.

Loving yourself is listening to your body's whispers, not shouts. Feeling tired? Recover. Feeling hungry? Eat. You're more likely to try that new healthy recipe or lace up your walking shoes because you know you deserve to feel good. You're more likely to choose activities you enjoy and ditch things that drain you.

With self-love, bumps in the road won't break you. You'll dust yourself off, kinder and stronger. This kindness makes you feel strong and energetic, giving you the power to keep going on your health journey, one kind decision at a time. Self-love allows you to give and receive love more openly.

And when you feel loved and supported by the people around you, it gives you a warm fuzzy feeling inside, right? That's not just happiness; it's a boost to your emotional health. Feeling loved helps you cope with stress, bounce back from challenges, and even feel less physical pain.

Respect is listening to your body's needs. It's about setting boundaries and saying what you need. When you respect your choices and boundaries, it makes you feel safe and valued. This sense of security lowers your anxiety and makes you feel more in control of your life.

Everyone has good days and some not-so-good days, healthy habits and not-so-healthy habits. Accepting yourself means not getting down on yourself for occasional setbacks but instead celebrating your progress and learning from your mistakes. When you accept yourself for who you are, it takes a huge weight off your shoulders. It's like giving yourself a big hug. It means understanding that you're not perfect, but you're worthy of love and happiness just the way you are. This self-acceptance helps you bounce back from setbacks and keeps you motivated on your health journey. You're not constantly trying to be someone you're not, which frees up energy for the things that truly matter.

Changing Your Life Isn't Difficult

Changing your life isn't difficult. The real challenge is changing yourself. Many people dream of better lives. They think, 'When I get that job, I'll be happier', or 'Once I have more money, everything will be better'. The truth is, if you don't change your habits and mindset, your life will stay the same.

It's not easy to change your life because it's hard to change yourself.

You keep pouring water into a leaky bucket, but it keeps leaking out. No matter how much water you add, the bucket stays empty. That's what happens when you try to change your life without changing yourself.

You see, your life is a reflection of you. If you're not happy on the inside, no amount of external change will make you truly happy. It's easier to wait for circumstances to change first, but circumstances won't change if you don't change first.

Waiting for the perfect moment or creating the perfect moment. The choice is all yours.

Anyone Can Change, But You Need to Want It

Anybody can change, but it starts with one important step: knowing why. When you understand the reason behind your need to change, you are opening the door to making that change happen.

You can change if you want to. You just need to know why you want to change.

It all begins with asking yourself, "Why do I want to change?" It's to live a healthier life, be happier, or improve relationships. Whatever the reason, it must be meaningful to you. This is your source of motivation. Knowing your why gives you strength and direction. It keeps you focused.

It is not enough to say you want to change. You need to truly want it, deep down. You can change, but it's not automatic. You need to *want* to change.

Once you know your why, you're ready to take the next step.

I have an exercise called 'complete the sentence'. It helps you discover why change is needed and why it matters. The idea behind this exercise is simple: when you know why to change, you're ready to start changing.

Here's how it works: fill in the blank, then write down why it really matters. Be honest with yourself as you write.

Write 4 meaningful reasons. If these reasons truly matter to you, they will drive your willingness to change.

I'll start first.

If I am fit and healthy, _I'll be more reliable for my family._

Why it matters? _I want to be there for my family, to help them, and to be emotionally present to keep a positive atmosphere at home._

Your Reason 1

If I am fit and healthy: _______________________

Why it matters?

Your Reason 2

If I am fit and healthy: ______________________________.

Why it matters?

Your Reason 3

If I am fit and healthy: ________________________.

Why it matters?

Your Reason 4

If I am fit and healthy: ________________________.

Why it matters?

Change For You, Not for Them

People feel anxious and insecure because they try to change just to fit into society. No matter how much you change, others will still have opinions. **Change** because it's what you want, not because others tell you to.

Change because you're not happy with yourself, not because others aren't happy with you.

Change because it makes you happy inside, not because you feel society wants you to.

Change because it matches your true values, not because it's someone else's idea of success.

Change because it allows you to explore and discover new passions, not just because others think it's good for you.

Don't change just because your situation has changed. *Change* so that you can change your situation.

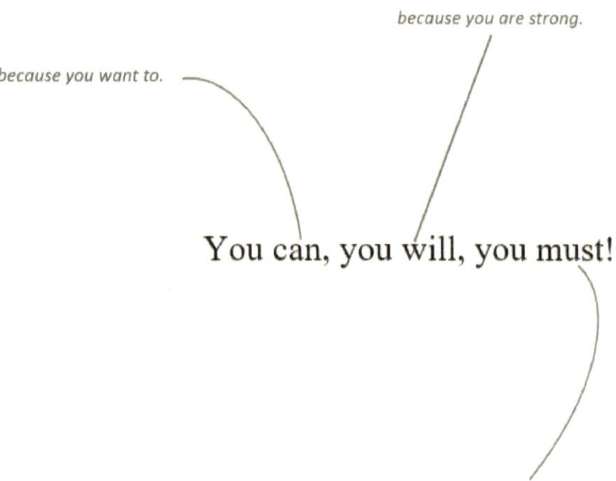
because you are strong.
because you want to.
You can, you will, you must!
because your life depends on it.

4

4 Simple Rules

You focus on work, family, and a million other things; life gets so busy that you forget the most important person - *yourself*. Your health and well-being are the foundation for everything else. When you feel good, you're happier, more productive at work, and more reliable for the people who depend on you. A healthy you is a happier you, a more reliable you, a better you, period.

A healthy you is a happier you, a more reliable you, a better you, period.

So why do you neglect yourself, the very thing that matters most? We hear the saying, "Health is wealth," but wealth gets mistaken for money and possessions.

'I don't have time to exercise,' 'Healthy food is too expensive.' But these are just excuses. You fear the effort, the change in routine. It's easier to stick with what's familiar, even if it's not doing you any favours.

The truth is you shy away from what's difficult. It's human nature to put off things that require effort. You have time to scroll through social media, but not to sweat it out? Again, it's all about perspective. You can change your life by changing your mind.

In this chapter, I want to share a few easy steps to a healthier you, steps I've used for years to maintain my own well-being.

Deep down, you want to feel healthy, happy, and look good. But because it seems hard, you settle for comfort. But true happiness comes from taking care of yourself.

Looking Good, Feeling Great

I'm happy. I'm confident. And yes, people often ask, "Shah, how do you stay in shape?"

Of course, some folks take a different approach. They say, "We only have one life, live it up!" But what exactly is 'living it up'? True enjoyment comes from feeling good about yourself, a sense of contentment and satisfaction. So, ask yourself, what brings you more joy – watching screens and admiring perfect lives or looking in the mirror and loving what you see? Isn't it more fulfilling to be the person others admire?

Simple, Slow and Steady

Most people give up because they make it too hard. They chase complex diets and intense workouts, only to get discouraged and quit. The key is to keep it simple, especially at the beginning. Consistency is what matters most. Just keep moving forward, even if it's at a slow pace.

Success is about taking lots of little steps over a long time, all moving in the right direction.

The reason you procrastinate on healthy habits is because of low self-esteem, fear, and not knowing where to start. That's why motivation is key. My goal is to give you something simple and easy to follow so you don't feel overwhelmed.

Strict diet plans and calorie counting are tough to stick with. They'll work for a short time, but then you burn out. It's better to take small steps regularly than try to do too much at once.

Getting healthy doesn't have to be complicated. Forget strict diets and intense workouts. It's all about small, simple steps.

Many people dream big and want to change everything at once. I have seen people out of shape who suddenly want to change; they starve themselves, spend hours at the gym, and try super hard for a little while, but it's just too much. They get sore, tired, and grumpy. Soon, they're back to their old habits.

The key is small steps! Big changes don't stick. Success, no matter what you're doing, is about taking lots of little steps over a long time, all moving in the right direction. Some people try to do too much too fast and then give up completely. Take small steps, keep moving forward, and you'll reach your goals.

Finding the Right Routine for Your Goals

In our quest for a healthier life, there's one key ingredient: the right daily habits. Whether you want to feel stronger, shed some pounds, or have more pep in your step, a good routine is your weapon.

If you hate what you do, it'll be tough to stick with it.

Figure out what exactly you want to achieve. Do you dream of running a marathon, fitting into your favourite jeans again, or just feeling less stressed? Once you know your destination, you can pick a path that leads you there.

Next, think about where you are now. If you haven't exercised much lately, don't jump straight into training for a weightlifting competition! Start with activities that fit your current fitness level to avoid getting hurt or discouraged.

Important thing? Finding a routine you actually enjoy. If you hate what you do, it'll be tough to stick with it. So, try different things, find what makes you happy, and watch the results come along.

A healthy life isn't just about physical results. It's about feeling good all around – mind, body, and spirit. No matter your specific health goal, my 4 simple rules will be your compass, guiding you on your journey to a happier, healthier you.

Forget the Fancy Stuff

Here's the deal: I don't follow a complicated diet plan or obsess over fat grams. Instead, I have a few basic rules that I've found work for me. Everyone's body is different, and everyone has different goals. But I can guarantee these rules will make a difference in your life. It will teach you discipline and self-control as long as you stick with it.

You don't need fancy equipment or flashy sneakers to be fit. You just need a little voice inside you that pushes you harder each day.

The world of health advice can feel like a jungle gym these days. New diets pop up faster than you can say 'kale', and workout routines promise beach bodies in a blink. But through all the trends, a few golden rules have stood the test of time. They're the building blocks for a healthy life; these rules will always be your friends on the path to a healthy life.

These aren't magic tricks but healthy habits that anyone can follow. 4 simple yet powerful rules that form the foundation of a healthy life, no matter what the latest trend might be. These are the simple rules I've followed for years, and I'm excited to share them with the world in hopes they'll make a positive difference in your life.

When people say you can't do it or it's too tough, those are their rules, not yours. Break their rules. But don't break your own rules.

Here are 4 simple rules that changed my life, and they can change yours, too.

Rule #1

Sweet Nothings, Oily Nothingness

We've all heard it a million times: 'Cut out sugar' feels like a broken record, but there's a reason this advice keeps popping up. Sugar, especially the kind hiding in processed foods, has become a major health concern.

The secret lies not in complete deprivation but in making smart swaps. Let's be honest: sugar is addictive. It triggers a feel-good response in our brains, making us crave more. But this constant sugar rush isn't doing your body any favours. It leads to weight gain and fatigue and even contributes to health problems down the line.

Refined sugar is like putting low-quality fuel in the tank. It gives you a temporary burst of energy, but it won't run smoothly for long.

Purchase a few really basic foods, like fruits, honey, and my personal favourite, dates, that readily substitute processed sugar. They are constantly accessible in my house. If I want to satisfy a sugar urge, I'll reach for a banana, a handful of dates, or even squeeze some honey into my mouth straight from the bottle; this stops the cravings right away.

Making changes doesn't have to be an all-or-nothing approach. Start small, swap out one sugary drink for water a day. Opt for fresh fruit instead of dessert a couple of nights a week. Slowly, you'll find that your taste buds adjust, and you start craving the natural sweetness of whole foods over processed sugar bombs.

By making these simple swaps, you're not just giving your taste buds a treat; you're giving your whole body a gift. You'll have more energy throughout the day, experience fewer cravings, and even feel lighter and healthier overall.

> *Every step away from sugar is a step towards a clearer mind and a stronger body.*

It's not about deprivation; it's about making conscious choices. There's still room for an occasional treat – a piece of birthday cake or a scoop of ice cream won't derail your progress. But by making natural sweetness your go-to choice, you'll be setting yourself up for a healthier, happier you.

Your Brain, Not Your Taste Buds

Taste buds tell us if something is yummy or yucky. But sometimes, even before a bite touches your tongue, your mind plays a trick. Have you ever heard someone rave about a delicious dessert, and suddenly you crave it, too? That's your mind at work! Your friend tells you about this incredible pie they just had. You listen, picturing the flaky crust and gooey filling. Your mind gets excited and starts to imagine the taste. It whispers, "Oh man, that sounds amazing!" The more you think about it, the stronger the feeling gets. Now, you can't stop picturing that pie, and your mouth starts to water.

This craving wasn't there before your friend spoke up. It's your mind, picturing the treat and making you want it more and more. If you hadn't paid so much attention to your friend's description, your brain wouldn't have had a chance to build up this craving. You would have simply said, "That's nice," and go about your day without a single thought of dessert. But because your mind got hooked on the idea, your body starts to feel like it needs that deliciousness right away.

This happens all the time. You see a commercial for a juicy burger, and the next thing you know, your stomach is rumbling. You walk past a bakery filled with fresh bread, and your willpower crumbles. Your mind has a strong influence over your desires and cravings.

The Real Deliciousness

That feeling when scrolling through social media and seeing a giant slice of cake, suddenly, your stomach starts to rumble. You see perfectly sculpted bodies, and a pang of insecurity hits. It's easy to fall for the idea that eating a certain food or looking a certain way equals feeling amazing and believing that happiness comes from outside. But nothing looks as good as feeling healthy feels.

Nothing looks as good as feeling healthy feels.

Sure, that dessert will be a temporary pleasure explosion in your mouth. But have you ever felt sluggish and heavy after a sugary treat? That's your body saying, "Whoa, that wasn't the best choice!"

The real deliciousness is not a fleeting pleasure from a sugary treat or having a six-pack abs. It's a deep sense of well-being that comes from taking care of yourself. It's feeling strong and confident. Feeling healthy is a real sweet treat.

And guess what? When you feel good inside, it shows on the outside. Your skin has a natural glow, your eyes sparkle with energy, and you move with confidence. That's a kind of beauty that comes from within, and it's much more powerful than any fleeting trend.

Seesaw

Let's be honest; there will be days when sugar cravings feel impossible to resist. That's okay! We all have them. The key is to balance things out. If you know you're going to indulge a bit one day, try to be extra good about saying no to sugar on other days. This way, it evens out in the long run.

Don't feel pressured to join the party scene just because there are sugary treats around. It's totally okay to politely decline. You're making a healthy choice for yourself. You're the boss of your body, and you get to decide what goes in it.

If you indulge in a sugary treat, try to make healthier choices for the rest of the day. It's like a seesaw; tilt it back towards healthy.

Muscles Turn Sugar into Power

The body's a marvellous machine, always working behind the scenes. Sugar, that sweet culprit we love, needs help getting used properly. Tiny sugar crystals floating in your bloodstream, unsure where to go. That's what happens when you don't have enough muscle mass.

Muscle acts like a sponge, soaking up sugar after a meal. This keeps your blood sugar levels steady. But without enough muscle, sugar builds up, and over time, this leads to health problems.

Here's how it works. When you eat sugar, the body releases insulin, a key that unlocks the door for sugar to enter your cells and give them energy. But without enough muscle, there aren't enough cells with unlocked doors ready to receive the sugar rush. All that unused sugar starts to cause problems.

Your muscles are hungry furnaces, always burning fuel to keep you moving. The more muscle you have, the more furnaces you have going, constantly chomping through sugar in your bloodstream. This helps keep your energy levels steady and even prevents sugar from building up too high. So, building strong muscles is like having a built-in sugar disposal system – you burn it faster, keeping you healthy and energised.

A healthy balance is important. Enjoy some sweet treats, but keep your body strong. That way, your body will use all the fuel it needs to keep you moving and feeling great!

Is Your Food Taking a Dip in Danger?

That feeling – the aroma of crispy fried food wafting through the air, tempting us with its golden promise. But before you dive headfirst into that basket of deep-fried goodness, take a moment to consider a different path. Those tempting treats come with a hidden cost to your health.

This simple rule has become the cornerstone of my healthy living journey – I avoid anything that's been deep-fried. Deep-fried delights increase your risk of heart disease, a condition that leads to serious health problems.

Think of your arteries as highways that carry blood throughout your body. Deep-fried foods are loaded with 2 types of villains: saturated fats and trans fats. These unhealthy fats act like sticky roadblocks, clogging those essential highways. Over time, this build-up makes it harder for your heart to pump blood efficiently, increasing your risk of heart disease, heart failure, heart attack, and stroke.

Be mindful of how your food is cooked. The next time you're faced with a tempting dish, take a moment to ask yourself, "Did this spend time submerged in a pool of oil?" If the answer is yes, it will be wise to explore other options.

> *Deep-fried out,*
> *vitality in.*

Changing habits takes time. You don't have to ditch your favourite fried foods overnight. It's about finding ways to enjoy delicious food without compromising your health. There's a whole world of flavour waiting to be explored beyond the deep fryer.

Your Body Shows You're a Winner

There are many things people show off to impress others. But the strongest symbol of success isn't a fancy car or expensive clothes. It's your own healthy body.

> *A fit body tells your story. It shows you have patience, discipline, resilience and self-control.*

A fit body tells your story. It shows you have patience; getting in shape takes time, and it's not a magic trick. It shows discipline and the power to push yourself even when it's tough. It shows resilience; you face setbacks, but you keep going. It shows the work ethic and effort you put in, day after day. It takes willpower to resist unhealthy temptations, showing you have self-control.

People respect someone who takes care of themselves. It shows you're strong, both physically and mentally. It's a message to the world that you are strong, determined, and in control. Invest in your health. It's the ultimate badge of honour.

Rule #2

Eat Like Clockwork

Life gets busy, schedules get thrown off, and suddenly, we're scrambling to eat dinner at midnight. But there is a way to eat that not only keeps you on track but also benefits your health. Time-restricted eating (TRE).

TRE is a way of eating that focuses on when you eat, not necessarily what you eat. It involves setting a specific window of time each day for your meals and snacks and then sticking to it. Studies suggest that TRE holds the key to a longer, healthier life. Researchers believe it could help lower the risk of serious illnesses like cancer and heart disease.

The Domino Effect

The thing is that when you miss a meal, it throws your whole day off track. Like dominoes falling over, one missed meal leads to another. A late breakfast pushes back lunch, which in turn makes dinner a late-night affair. This disrupted eating pattern wreaks havoc on your body.

My Simple Trick for Staying on Schedule

Simplify your eating, amplify your living.

I know life can be hectic, especially in the mornings when everyone's rushing out the door. That's why I have a simple rule for myself: if I can't finish my meal within my set time frame, I skip it and have a light snack on hand to hold me over until the next scheduled meal. It sounds strict, but it works.

Finding Your Mealtime Rhythm

Everyone's body is different, so the ideal TRE window will vary from person to person. But for me, it looks like this:

Breakfast before 8 am: I love a good breakfast, so I make sure to wake up early enough to enjoy it. This encourages me to get a good night's sleep, creating a healthy routine.

Lunch before 1 pm: This gives my body enough time to digest and feel energised for the rest of the afternoon.

Dinner at least an hour before bed: This gives my body time to wind down and prepare for sleep, which is crucial for overall health.

Following this routine has helped me develop self-control and better time-management skills. I know when my body needs food, and I plan my day accordingly.

The Power of Healthy Snacks

Of course, there will be times when you can't finish a meal on time or something unexpected throws your schedule off. That's okay! But to avoid unhealthy late-night snacking, I always keep a stash of healthy snacks on hand. These snacks tide you over until your next meal without derailing your TRE routine.

Following a TRE plan isn't just about restricting your eating window – it's about building self-control and time management skills. By planning your meals and sticking to a schedule, you're essentially taking control of your health and well-being. Experiment and find what works best for you and your body.

TRE is a flexible approach. You can adjust the time window to fit your lifestyle. The key is to find what works for you and stick with it as much as possible.

With a little planning and discipline, you can make TRE work for you. It may not be a complete 'no' to food outside your window, but it's a conscious choice to prioritise a healthy and well-timed eating pattern. So, set your internal clock and feel your best.

Most Important Meal of The Day

Need a hearty breakfast to start your day strong? Forget the old ideas about which meal is most important. A healthy meal, whether it's in the morning, afternoon, or evening, packed with good stuff, keeps you energised, focused, and feeling your best.

The key is to choose nutritious foods throughout the day, no matter what meal it is.

Rule #3

Move Your Body, Move Your Mood

The word 'exercise' — it can strike fear in the hearts of even the most well-intentioned people. Images of crowded gyms, clanging weights, and gruelling workouts come to mind.

Exercise means any physical activity that helps you stay healthy and fit. It doesn't have to involve expensive gym memberships, intimidating weightlifting, or pricey trainers (although there's a place for all of those things if that's what motivates you!).

Fitness fuels confidence.

A brisk walk in the park, a refreshing swim in the pool, or a bike ride along a scenic path — these are all forms of exercise! You can get your body moving without breaking the bank or leaving the comfort of your neighbourhood.

Beyond the Physical

The benefits of exercise go far beyond just a toned physique. Exercise is a powerful tool for transforming your mind, mood, and overall attitude.

As the saying goes, "Exercise not only changes your body, it changes your mind, your attitude and your mood." It's true! Physical activity has been shown to boost energy levels, reduce stress and anxiety, and even improve sleep quality. So, the next time you're feeling sluggish or down, put your shoes on and get moving – your mind and body will thank you!

Workout for the feeling, not the look.

While the idea of exercise seems daunting at first, incorporating it into your life is surprisingly easy. Don't try to go from a couch potato to a marathon runner overnight. Begin with short, manageable bursts of activity – a 15-minute walk every day is a great place to start. Gradually increase the duration and intensity as you get fitter.

Schedule your workouts in your calendar like any other appointment. This helps treat exercise with the importance it deserves and prevents it from getting pushed aside.

It's tempting to fall into unhealthy habits or skip workouts, especially when life gets busy. But remember, consistency is key. Don't get discouraged if you miss a workout here and there; just get back on track the next day. Exercise shouldn't feel like punishment. Find something you genuinely look forward to, and you'll be more likely to stick with it.

There will be bumps along the way, but the key is consistency, not perfection. Start slowly, find activities you enjoy, and don't give up. This is just the beginning of your journey. Explore different activities, find what works for you, and most importantly, have fun!

Me Time

I've heard it too many times: "I'm just too busy to work out." Life gets hectic, schedules jam-packed, and suddenly, taking care of ourselves seems like a luxury we can't afford. The bitter truth is, if you can't make 30 minutes for your own well-being, you've messed up in your life.

If you can't make 30 minutes for your own well-being, you've messed up in your life.

Now, I'm not judging. We all have our struggles. Life gets busy. Work, family, errands – it all piles up. But wouldn't you rather navigate that busy life with a clear head and a smile on your face? If you neglect your health, everything else becomes harder. You get tired easily, can't focus, and even get sick more often. Think of those 30 minutes as a way to recharge your batteries. You'll have more energy for everything else in your life, and you'll feel better overall.

Let's be real, 30 minutes isn't a lifetime. It's less than an episode of your favourite show. It's shorter than most commutes and definitely less time than you spend scrolling through social media.

You don't need to become a gym rat. We're not talking about spending hours lifting weights or running on a treadmill (unless that's your jam, of course!). There are tonnes of other ways to get moving.

You could even break it down into smaller chunks – 15 minutes in the morning for some stretches or yoga and 15 minutes before bed for a calming walk.

The key is to find something you actually enjoy. If you hate running, don't force yourself to do it. There's an exercise out there for everyone; you just have to find what clicks for you.

Investing 30 minutes in yourself is like investing in the best possible version of yourself. Schedule those 30 minutes just like you would any other important appointment. You're worth the investment.

The best company I could ever ask for is myself. You're never truly alone when you have your own incredible spirit by your side.

And once you start feeling the benefits of regular exercise, you may even find yourself craving those 30 minutes. It becomes a time to clear your head, de-stress, and feel accomplished. You'll find yourself looking forward to those little pockets of 'me time'.

Stressed & Too Tired

Many people with jobs throw their hands up and say, "Exercise? No time! My job is too much!" But exercise is your stress-busting superhero! Exercise is a chance to take a break, to focus on your body and move your muscles with glee. It lets your mind unwind and forget the daily worries.

When you move your body, it releases happy chemicals that fight stress and make you feel fantastic. It's like a natural mood booster. Sure, you might be tired after a long day, but a short burst of exercise is a magic trick. You'll feel more energised and focused.

Ditch the 'too stressed for exercise' thought! It's like giving up your strongest weapon against the daily grind. Exercise isn't a burden; it's a stress-busting treasure chest! Find activities you enjoy. Make it fun, make it short, but make it happen.

Real Challenge

Anyone can tell you the hardest part of exercise is the workout itself. Pushing your muscles, getting sweaty, feeling that burn – that's tough. But I'll let you in on a little secret: the real challenge is way before you even start.

> *The real challenge is way before you even start. It's the voice in your head.*

It's that voice in your head, "Just 5 more minutes," or "I'm too tired today, I'll start tomorrow." That's where the battle starts. Most people don't give up on exercise because it's too hard – they give up on that internal fight to get going. That voice is what makes people give up, not the actual workout. They give up on the battle before it starts.

Once you trick your mind, the rest falls into place. Your body wakes up; the endorphins kick in.

Perfect Time to Exercise

Your body craves movement, just like it craves food. You wouldn't skip a meal, so don't skip exercise. Find a time that works for you, even if it changes day to day. The most important thing is to get your body moving.

The more you move your body, the more your body will move for you.

Forget about the perfect time. Be flexible, and listen to your body. If mornings are crazy, squeeze it in later. Afternoons swamped? No worries, hit it after work. Just get moving whenever you can. Even a short workout is better than no workout at all. The key is consistency, not the clock.

Monkey See, Monkey Do

You've probably heard this saying "Monkey see, monkey do." Well, sometimes it seems like that's all some people are doing! They watch others lift weights or run on machines, then copy them without a clue.

Just because someone else is lifting heavy weights doesn't mean that's the best thing for you. Everyone's body is different, and everyone has different reasons for wanting to get fit. Maybe you want to tone up and get more flexible, or you just want to have more energy to keep up with the kids. Whatever your goal, blindly following others won't get you there. What works for them won't necessarily work for you.

Figure out what you want to achieve. Do you want to build muscle? Lose weight? Feel stronger and more energetic? Once you know your goal, you can find the exercises that will help you reach it.

Fantastic 4

Have you ever wondered why some people seem to build muscle easily while others struggle to gain weight? Our bodies come in all shapes and sizes, and that's perfectly normal! There are actually 4 main body types that can help you understand how your body naturally tends to store fat and muscle.

Ectomorphs are naturally thin individuals. They have a lean build with narrow shoulders and long limbs. They find it difficult to gain weight, both muscle and fat.

Endomorphs have rounder bodies and tend to store fat more easily. They have naturally broad shoulders and hips. Weight gain, both muscle and fat, comes easily to endomorphs.

Mesomorphs are the athletic bunch. They have a naturally muscular build and tend to gain muscle and lose fat more easily than the other 2 types. They have broad shoulders and a narrow waist.

Finally, there's the **mixed type**. This is like a choose-your-own-adventure for bodies! Most people actually fall into this category, a blend of 2 or even all 3! You have an ectomorph's thin build but can build muscle like an endomorph. Or perhaps you have an endomorph's curves but an easy time losing weight like a mesomorph.

There's no single 'best' body type. Each one is unique and awesome in its own way. The best workout routine is the one you enjoy and that fits your body. Don't compare yourself to others - embrace your amazing shape and find the exercises that make you feel strong and happy! So, don't just copy what others are doing. Consider your body type and what your goals are.

4 Essential Workouts

We know exercise is good for us, but did you know there are different ways to move your body that target different things? It's like having a toolbox full of workout tools, and each tool helps you build a stronger you!

You'll not always love your workout, but you'll love the way you feel afterward.

Endurance. It's all about keeping your heart pumping and your lungs happy. It helps you last longer during exercise and in everyday life, like climbing stairs without getting winded.

Strength training. Lifting weights or doing push-ups. Strength workouts make your muscles bigger and stronger, which helps you lift heavier things, improve your posture, and even burn more calories during recovery. Strong muscles are like superheroes for your everyday life!

Balance. Staying steady on your feet – that's balance. Balance exercises help you stay stable and prevent falls, which is super important as we get older. It improves your coordination, making you more graceful and sure-footed in all your activities.

Flexibility. It's all about stretching and bending. Stretching your arms and reaching for your toes or twisting your torso. Flexibility workouts help your muscles and joints move freely, which improves your range of motion and makes everyday tasks easier. Plus, they feel great and help prevent injuries.

What are the best workout routines? A well-rounded workout routine has a bit of everything to keep your body strong, balanced, and ready to take on anything!

Effort Over Hours

Going to the gym for hours every day, sweating and lifting weights, hoping to transform your body quickly? Spending long hours at the gym won't magically make you brand new. It's not about the quantity of time you spend working out but the quality of your effort.

> *It's not about the quantity of time you spend working out but the quality of your effort.*

It's the dedication and focus you put into each workout session that truly makes a difference. You could do a short, intense workout with full dedication and see better results than hours of half-hearted exercise.

Instead of counting the hours, focus on giving your best during your workout. Push yourself a little harder, and challenge your limits. That's where the real transformation happens – in the moments where you push through the discomfort and give it your all.

It's not about the length of your workout sessions but the intensity of your effort that will bring you closer to your fitness goals. Quality over quantity, every time.

Fuel, Recover, Move: Back to Basics

Everyone wants that magic solution, the secret shortcut to a better life. But it's the simple things that pack the biggest punch. Focus on the basics: good food that fuels your body, enough sleep to recharge, and exercise that gets you moving.

> *It's hard work, but it's clear work.*

When you cloud your mind with unnecessary complexity, you create barriers where none exist. When you focus on the basics, you cut through the clutter and confusion. No more fads, no more frustration. Just steady progress, step by step. It's hard work, but it's clear work.

Now, the 4th rule I am about to share may seem a bit unusual, but it's incredibly powerful for your health. It's something that people don't connect with health, but it's important. It's a powerful force that will transform your health journey in unexpected ways.

Rule #4

Inner Peace

Finding peace inside is the best health you can have. Gratitude brings inner peace. It's a secret ingredient in a recipe for a healthier life. Overlooked when discussing health, where the spotlight usually shines on diet, exercise, and sleep. However, gratitude is arguably the most powerful catalyst for well-being.

I am thankful for everything I had in life; I am thankful for everything I have in life, and I am thankful for everything I will have in life.

When you practise gratitude, everything shifts. It's like putting on a pair of glasses that make everything look better. When you are grateful, your whole view of life improves. Every day becomes brighter, and life feels more joyful and full.

By fostering gratitude, you reduce stress—one of the major culprits behind many chronic diseases. Gratitude shifts your focus away from problems and deficiencies, helping to quell anxiety and boosting mental health. It enhances sleep quality, strengthens the immune system, and lowers blood pressure. It's like a free, natural therapy, free from side effects, that enhances your body's resilience and vitality.

Gratitude is like a battery for the soul that keeps you charged with positive energy. When you are grateful, you focus less on what you lack and more on what you have. This helps you feel more content and less anxious.

And the most compelling thing is that it's so easy to do. All you have to do is say these words: I am thankful for everything I had in life; I am thankful for everything I have in life, and I am thankful for everything I will have in life. They cost nothing, yet the rewards they bring are priceless.

Gratitude is something we all naturally know how to express. Remember the moment you got that well-deserved promotion at work? There was that burst of thankfulness, a genuine appreciation for the acknowledgement of your hard work. Or think back to when you received a pay raise, a moment of validation; you couldn't help but feel grateful. The day you met your partner, your heart was full of thanks, knowing you'd found someone special. The pride and joy when you sat behind the wheel of your very first car, knowing your hard work had tangible results.

As I write this, I realise just how often we overlook the practice of gratitude. We can never show it enough. Gratitude is something you already know how to show. From now on, just try to remember to do it all the time.

It is quite possibly the most valuable investment you can make for your well-being. A zero-cost path to a healthier, happier life.

There are many ways to express gratitude and countless things to appreciate. Here's what I do: *When I wake up, I sit up in bed, place my feet on the floor, close my eyes, and say, "Thank you for giving me another day to express gratitude, seek forgiveness, and set things right. Thank you for the breath I have." Then I rise and say, "Thank you for giving me the strength and energy to stand on my own."*

And off I go, starting my day. It only takes a minute, but starting the day with this tone and positive energy makes the entire day feel more organised and productive. I start to notice the positives in everything.

This is just my way, but you can find your own way to do it. Just make sure you do it.

These 4 simple rules will make a big difference in how you feel. Following these rules is like building a solid foundation for a healthy life. You'll learn to take care of yourself and keep going, even when it's hard.

The more we have of something, the less we seem to appreciate it. Happiness isn't having more but instead appreciating what you already have.

Think of these rules as a map to feeling good and balanced in all parts of your life. By making them a habit, you're setting yourself up for long-lasting health and energy. Each rule helps you feel better in all ways, both inside and out. So, I really hope you'll try them and stick with them. By following these rules, you're not just getting healthier; you're learning to respect yourself and be strong.

The more you follow these rules, the more you're investing not just in your body but also in how well you know yourself and your own power. They're like lighthouses showing you the way to complete well-being. They'll help you appreciate your body, mind, and spirit. So, try your best to follow them and keep your promise to yourself.

By making these rules a habit, you're building a path to lasting health and energy. Stay committed, listen to your body, and take care of yourself. You're not just changing your health; you're making your life more meaningful, energetic, and strong. Just don't break your own rules.

A Day Late, But Still a Dream

A friend of mine really loved BMW convertibles. He always said, "One day, I'll buy this car for myself." Whenever he saw one on the road, he felt so happy and would always say, "I will own it one day." He worked very hard for it, and finally, on his 38th birthday, he booked his favourite car. He told the showroom he wanted it delivered on his birthday.

But, for some reason, the showroom couldn't deliver it on his birthday—they delivered it the next day. The excitement of receiving the car wasn't apparent on his face. He was upset and unhappy because the car wasn't delivered on the day he wanted. Despite having waited five years and worked so hard to get it, he was disappointed.

Sometimes, life doesn't give us what we want exactly the way we want it, but it does give us what we wish for if we really deserve it. Don't spoil the enjoyment of having it just because you didn't get it on your terms. Be thankful that you got what you desired. Be grateful—no matter how, where, or when you receive it.

Even if your dream comes true a day late, it's still your dream; it still means you've made it. Your dreams are valid, no matter when they come true.

Now, before doing anything else, pause for a moment, no matter where you are—on your couch, at a coffee shop, or by the beach. Just stop and do this. I want you to close your eyes, take a deep breath, and say 'thank you' for the mere fact that you are breathing.

Now, think of 4 things you are grateful for. It could be anything. Maybe remember the first time you met your partner. Or perhaps recall a delicious meal you enjoyed today.

As you think about these moments, really feel the emotions that arise. Those feelings are your strength. They are the ones that make you strong—emotionally, mentally, and physically. These emotions are like a tonic for your well-being, nourishing you in a way nothing else can. Practising gratitude makes you resilient, healthier, and more content.

Now I want you to write those 4 things that you thought about. Because when you write, you see them right in front of your eyes. When you put them on paper, they become more than thoughts; they become visible and real. Writing makes these moments tangible. You can revisit them anytime, feeling the same joy and gratitude. Trust me, I know the power of words. They have a way of making things clearer and more meaningful.

First, write down what you're thankful for. Then, add a word that describes how you felt while thinking about it, like 'happy' or 'excited'. Finally, end by writing 'thank you'.

I am grateful for:

I am grateful for:

I am grateful for:

I am grateful for:

Real People, Real Style

I once saw a coworker excitedly ordering clothes online, only to mutter later, "I wonder how they look on normal people?" It's true, those model pictures are deceiving! Super skinny figures and perfect lighting make you think looking good is only possible for models and celebrities, but that's not quite right.

Sure, models often have a specific body type. But that doesn't mean you can't look and feel fantastic in your own skin. Looking great isn't about replicating a model's figure. It's about feeling confident and healthy in your own skin. When you focus on taking care of yourself, you naturally start to radiate a healthy glow.

Sure, some clothes look different on you than on a model, but that's because you're a real person, not a perfectly posed picture! The best outfit is the one that makes you feel fantastic, and that confidence is more attractive than any filter.

Never Quit

Life is a long, winding road. Sometimes, it's smooth and sunny; other times, it's bumpy and filled with rain. There will be hills that seem impossible to climb and valleys that feel bottomless. But there's only one rule for navigating this road – never quit.

Quitting is like giving up on a delicious meal halfway through – you'll never experience the full satisfaction.

When faced with a challenge, the easy option is to throw in the towel and walk away. But quitting is like giving up on a delicious meal halfway through – you'll never experience the full satisfaction. Persistence, on the other hand, is the key that unlocks the doors of success and happiness.

Life is full of setbacks. You might not get the job you wanted, you might fail a test, or you might have a fight with a friend. These setbacks are inevitable, but they are not the end of the story. They are simply bumps on the road, not roadblocks.

So, what do you do when you face a setback? You pick yourself up. You dust yourself off. You learn from your mistakes and keep moving forward. Even the most successful people in the world have faced setbacks. The difference is that they never let those setbacks define them. They used them as stepping stones to reach even greater heights.

Quitting is contagious. When you give up on something, it sends a message to yourself and others that things are too difficult. But persistence is contagious, too! When you keep going, you inspire those around you to do the same. You become a beacon of hope, showing them that anything is possible.

Life isn't always fair. There will be times when you feel like you're putting in all the effort and getting nowhere. But persistence isn't about immediate results. It's about the long-term journey. It's about the small victories along the way. It's about knowing that every step you take, no matter how small, brings you closer to your goals.

When you have a clear purpose, it becomes easier to never quit.

A river never stops flowing, even when it meets a large rock in its path. The water doesn't give up; it finds a way around the obstacle. It carves a new channel, flows over the top, or goes underground. The river keeps moving because it has a purpose – to reach the ocean.

You need to have a purpose in life, a dream that keeps you motivated, even on the toughest days. It could be anything: living a healthy lifestyle, becoming a great athlete, starting a business, or being the best version of yourself. When you have a clear purpose, it becomes easier to never quit because you know why you're pushing yourself in the first place.

So, the next time you feel like giving up, remember the one rule of life: never quit. Keep going, keep fighting, and never lose sight of your dreams. The journey may be long and winding, but the rewards of persistence are worth every step.

Rest is for the Grave, Recovery is for the Living

Recover, not rest. Rest is just staying put, like a rock. Recovery is like taking a deep breath before the next climb. Sleep? It's recovery fuel for the battles tomorrow brings. Relaxing? That's your brain recharging for the next move. Rest is for the motionless, the finished. We are built to recover, to gasp for air and rise again.

> *Rest is for those who have finished their climb. We, the living, are all about recovery.*

Rest is a promise for the quiet of the grave. We are alive, and that means we recover endlessly until our final rest. Recover, yes, always. But rest? Not until the dirt naps on top of you. Until then, keep yourself prepped for what's to come.

I've deliberately avoided the word 'rest' in the book. Rest is for those who have finished their climb. We, the living, are all about recovery, the constant preparation for the next ascent.

Recharge

Life is a journey, not a sprint. There will be mountains to climb and valleys to cross, scorching deserts and stormy seas. Sometimes, the weight on your shoulders will feel unbearable, the path ahead blurry with doubt. Your muscles ache, your breath comes heavily, and a voice whispers in your ear, "Give up. It's too hard."

Recover. Yes, recover. It's not a weakness; it's a necessity. Take a deep breath, let your body unwind. Let the worries of the journey ease away for a moment. Sleep under the stars and feel the cool earth beneath you.

Recover, but never stop dreaming, never stop believing. Recovery is not the absence of movement but a preparation for the next step. It's a chance to gather your strength to find your focus. So, let your body and mind find solace in the pause. But never let the fire within you die. Keep your eyes on the horizon, and when you're ready, rise again and continue your journey. The greatest discoveries are made just beyond the point where you think you can't go any further.

The Simple Truth

What's more important for fitness? Exercise, food, or supplements? The simple truth is, "It's consistency and discipline."

You see, sticking to your routine and staying focused are the keys to success in getting fit. It's not just about sweating in the gym or eating well for a day. It's about doing it every day, even when you don't feel like it. Showing up and putting in the work, no matter what. It's about making small progress every day, even if it's just a little bit. Discipline is about saying no to temptations that derail your goals.

So, when you ask me about workouts, diet, or supplements, I say it's all about staying true to your plan and being committed. That's how you'll see real results and become the best version of yourself.

Is Waking Up Early a Sign of Discipline?

Someone once told me waking up early doesn't show you are disciplined. I totally disagree, and here's why that idea misses the mark!

Each time you listen to your disciplined self, you become stronger.

Waking up early in the morning is a powerful habit. Waking up early is a choice, and it's a hard one. Your bed is warm and inviting, and it feels so good to sleep more. But when you decide to leave that comfort and meet the rising sun, you are showing discipline.

Discipline is about making the right choices, even when it's tough. It is about not giving in to the lazy voice in your head that says, "Sleep for a while more. You don't need to get up." Choosing to ignore that voice takes strength and persistence.

Being disciplined is about controlling those little voices in your head every day. Discipline means doing what you know is right. Each time you listen to your disciplined self, you become stronger. When you wake up early, you show yourself that you are in control, not the lazy feeling. You have decided to own your morning and make it your victory.

So yes, waking up early shows discipline. It's about making a difficult choice and sticking with it. It helps you win over your temptations, making it easier to make good choices in other parts of your life, too.

When you wake up early, it's just you, and this is the time to focus on what you need to do, understanding your purpose and your reasons for being here without any distractions. You don't need coffee to kickstart your day; you just need to wake up and connect with yourself. Tuning into yourself not only moves you, it changes you.

For many, the thought of waking up early feels impossible, so they choose not to even try. Waking up early while the world sleeps provides a unique perspective. It allows you to solidify your plans, goals, and dreams in your mind. Once you achieve that clarity, you can realize them in reality.

Whatever becomes clear in your head, you can hold it in your hand.

Rising early provides you with peace, quiet, and solitude, allowing you to focus on self-conditioning and preparation. It helps you connect with yourself, get into a rhythm, and perform at your peak. By minimizing distractions, you achieve a sharp focus on what matters most and gain a clear vision of your future.

From Effort to Excellence

Hard work is important. It's the sweat, the effort, the pushing ourselves that gets things done. But what if there was a secret ingredient that made all that hard work even more effective?

Discipline is a muscle that gets stronger with use.

You are sprinting towards a finish line. You push yourself to the limit, muscles burning, lungs screaming. That's hard work, giving it your all in a burst of effort. But what if, halfway through, you stumble and fall? The finish line seems further away than ever.

This is where discipline steps in. It's the steady hand that keeps you moving forward, even when the going gets tough. It's the difference between a quick burst of energy and achieving a long-term goal.

When you wake up feeling energised, ready to tackle the day, with a body that feels strong and capable, it's the power of discipline working its magic on your health.

We all face moments of weakness. That extra slice of cake calling your name or the urge to skip a workout for a movie. This is where discipline shines. It's the inner voice that reminds you of your long-term goals and helps you resist short-term temptations.

Hard work helps you push through a tough workout session, but it won't always win against cravings. Discipline acts like a wise adviser, guiding you towards healthy choices. It empowers you to build a healthy lifestyle, not just by working hard but also by making smart choices. It's waking up early to exercise, even if you're tired, or choosing a healthy meal even when surrounded by tempting treats. These consistent choices, repeated over time, are the building blocks of success.

Discipline helps you stay focused even when motivation wanes. There will be days when you don't feel like working towards your goals. But discipline keeps you going, reminding you of your 'why' – the reason you started this journey in the first place.

We face challenges on the road to success. Distractions, temptations, and setbacks throw us off track. Hard work will get you past one obstacle, but discipline is like a skilled rider taming a wild horse. It allows you to anticipate challenges and navigate them with focus and control.

It equips you with the tools to overcome those obstacles. It teaches you to resist distractions, find healthy alternatives to temptations, and bounce back stronger after setbacks. This resilience is key to achieving any long-term goal.

Discipline is a muscle that gets stronger with use. The more you practice, the easier it becomes to make it a part of your everyday life. Discipline is self-control, and by building self-control, you can unlock the potential to achieve anything you set your mind to.

> *Discipline is choosing your life rather than just letting it happen to you.*

If you control your thoughts, you control your life. How do you control your thoughts? By practising discipline.

Knowledge to Action

Knowledge is power, that's for sure. Filling your head with knowledge is fantastic! Books, podcasts, lectures – all these things open doors to new ideas. But knowledge by itself won't change anything. It's like collecting delicious recipes without ever stepping into the kitchen.

The real adventure begins when you take action. You use those tools, follow the map, and take that first step. That's when the knowledge clicks. You learn by doing, by facing challenges and seeing how your plans work in the real world.

So, while reading and listening are important, don't let them become an excuse to stay put. True learning comes from taking action. It's about putting what you've learned into practice. Whether it's trying a new skill or changing a small habit, doing something with your knowledge is what makes it stick.

The 4 Fears We Live By

People care deeply about 4 main things: money, status, popularity, and power. These are the things that shape our lives and choices. Many people worry about losing their jobs. This fear pushes them to get up early, rush to the office, and work hard, even in jobs they hate. Why? It is simple. They are afraid of losing their job because losing a job means losing money, status, popularity, and power.

People prioritise what they fear losing, yet all too often, health falls by the wayside.

Money is security. Without it, people worry about not being able to pay bills or afford daily needs. They fear what will happen if they fall behind. Along with money, there is status. This is how people see you in society. Those with high status enjoy respect and admiration.

Popularity is another concern. People want to be liked and accepted. They fear that losing their job will lead to losing friends and social connections. Power is the last piece. It gives people control over their lives and decisions. Losing a job can take away this power, making them feel weak and helpless.

Now, how often do we pause to consider, "What if I face a health crisis?" For many, this thought is pushed aside until it's too late.

People only care and value things they are afraid of losing. Sadly, health is not one of those valuable things for many people.

Live, Laugh, and Let Go

One day, I skipped my workout to hang out with friends. On our way, we grabbed a doughnut. Soon after, I felt guilty. My mind was racing, worrying about the missed workout and the doughnut. I kept thinking, "Oh no, I ate extra calories and didn't exercise." I was stressed so much that I couldn't relax and enjoy my time with friends. It was a lot of stress over a small thing. The stress over missing my workout and eating the doughnut was worse than the doughnut itself. It's important to take care of our health, but we shouldn't obsess over every little thing. Being hard on ourselves does more harm than good. We all need a break from our routine sometimes, so just enjoy it. You can always return to your routine the next day.

*When you try to control
everything, you enjoy
nothing. Sometimes,
you just need to relax,
breathe, let go and live
in the moment.*

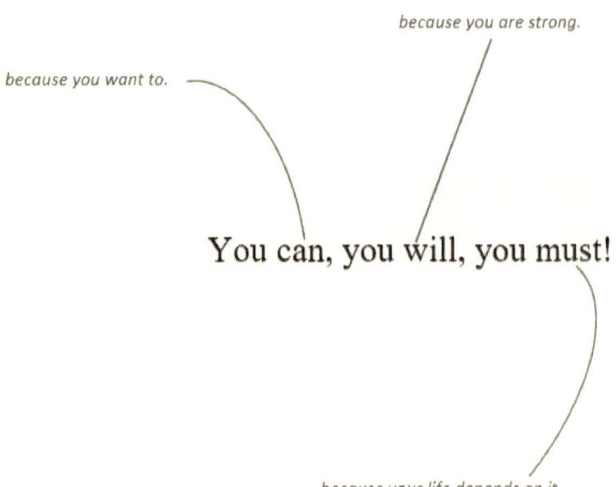
because you are strong.
because you want to.
You can, you will, you must!
because your life depends on it.

The Magic Drink

A few years ago, my friend had a problem with kidney stones. Kidney stones are small, hard deposits that form in the kidneys and can be very painful. My friend was experiencing discomfort because of these kidney stones. He decided to visit the doctor to seek help.

The doctor suggested a special drink that my friend now calls a 'magic drink.' This drink supposedly had the power to help with kidney stones and provide relief. The doctor spoke about this drink in a way that made it sound incredible. He highlighted the benefits of the drink and made it seem almost too good to be true.

The doctor's words sparked a flicker of hope in my friend's eyes. My friend had never heard of it before, and he wasn't sure what to think. But the doctor spoke with such confidence, like a wise old wizard explaining a secret spell. Could this simple drink truly be the answer to his troubles? The idea was almost too good to be believed, but it was enough to make my friend curious. He had to give it a try.

Days turned into weeks as my friend diligently consumed the magic drink as recommended by the doctor. He started to notice some subtle changes in how he felt. The discomfort from the kidney stones seemed to be easing, and my friend's overall well-being appeared to be improving. Could it be possible that the magic drink was actually working its wonders?

As time passed, my friend's condition continued to improve. The kidney stones that had caused him such discomfort were gradually reducing in size. The frequent bouts of pain he had experienced before were becoming less severe. My friend's energy levels were increasing, and he felt more like his old self again.

The simple drink had worked wonders for my friend's health and well-being. Intrigued, I decided to delve deeper. I started researching this magic elixir to understand how it could fit into my own health journey.

My research journey took me through conversations with nutritionists and dives into the world of health benefits. After gathering information, I decided to give it a try. I made a change to my own morning routine. Each day, I started my day with a simple concoction: a teaspoon of this magic elixir mixed with 500ml of water, all consumed on an empty stomach. It wasn't exactly love at first sip, but I found I could tolerate the taste.

It's a quick and easy addition to my day, and the results have been impressive. I have noticed a positive impact on my overall health. What was this mysterious potion, you ask? Believe it or not, it wasn't some fancy supplement or rare ingredient. It was *'apple cider vinegar'*. While it may sound ordinary, the effects have been nothing short of extraordinary. Since incorporating this magic drink into my routine, I've noticed positive changes.

One of the most noticeable transformations was a reduction in unwanted body fat. It wasn't a dramatic shift overnight, but a steady whittling down that left me feeling lighter and more energised. This fat loss wasn't just about aesthetics; it was a sign that my body was functioning more efficiently.

Another remarkable benefit was a noticeable boost in my metabolism. This internal furnace seemed to burn brighter, allowing me to process food more effectively. I no longer felt sluggish after meals, and my energy levels remained stable throughout the day.

But the most fascinating discovery was the profound impact on my gut health. It turns out that this hidden world within us plays a critical role in our overall well-being. As I started drinking 'apple cider vinegar', I noticed a significant improvement in digestion. Gone were the days of discomfort and bloating. My gut seemed to be working in harmony, efficiently extracting nutrients from food and keeping everything running smoothly. It seems the doctor was right after all – this simple drink is truly magical!

4 Silent Forces

Bonus tips for leading a happy, healthy, and successful life: Remember these 4 rules to succeed in any area of your life.

Work, Don't Speak

First, act; then achieve; and finally, announce.

Do your work in quiet. Don't shout about your plans from the rooftop. Don't tell everyone what you're going to do. Just do it. When you finish, they'll know. The accomplishment itself will be the announcement.

Work, Don't Show

Under the radar, over the top.

Don't try to prove to people that you're smart. It's a waste of energy. It's even better if they think you're not. Let them underestimate you. It gives you room to surprise them. True intelligence isn't about showing off; it's about getting things done. It's about understanding the world around you. You don't need a parade to celebrate that.

Act, Don't React

You are not obligated to respond. Not every battle requires a verbal defence, and not every insult deserves your energy.

When someone speaks against you, remember you don't always have to reply. Let your actions speak louder, proving them wrong without saying a word. Silence can be your strongest answer. Show your worth through what you do. Your life is your message. Make each moment of strength and success show everyone how strong you are. A silent slap, backed by potent actions, often hurts deeper than a loud one.

Speak to Open Ears

Talk where it matters.

Don't waste your breath trying to explain things to people who aren't ready to listen. Some people have their minds made up. Some people aren't open to new ideas. You can't force them. Save your words for those who are willing to hear them.

Final Words

We live in a time of amazing technology. We have gadgets that fit in our pockets and connect us to the whole world. We can order food with a tap, track our sleep with a watch, and even get medical advice online. But when it comes to our health, the most important things are still pretty simple and don't require anything fancy.

The foundation of good health is built on low-tech habits.

Think about it like this: your body is a machine. To run well, it needs a few key things: good fuel, regular maintenance, and time to recover. That's all there is to it! The high-tech stuff can be helpful for monitoring and fine-tuning, but the foundation of good health is built on low-tech habits.

It's not about complicated diets or fancy ingredients. A juicy apple is better than a sugary candy bar, and a bowl of rice is better than a bag of chips. Of course, there's room for treats now and then! Just like adding sprinkles to your healthy sundae. The sprinkles are fun, but you wouldn't want them to be the only thing in the bowl.

Good health doesn't require expensive gadgets or complicated routines. It's about making small, sustainable changes to your daily life. Don't try to overhaul your entire life overnight. Start with one or 2 small changes and gradually add more as they become habits. Small changes add up.

The Question Holding You Back

The world rushes by so fast that it's easy to get stuck saying, "Why now? Why me?" We wonder why things happen when they do and worry we're not ready. That worry makes us stressed and scared.

Many people focus on why they can't do something, not on why they should.

Instead of asking, "Why now?" ask yourself, "Why not give this a shot? Why not step outside my comfort zone?" This way, problems become stepping stones, and mistakes become lessons.

Many people focus on why they can't do something, not why they should. This keeps them stuck and prevents them from living their best life.

A common excuse is not having enough time, money, or help. But there's never a perfect time. Life is full of surprises and bumps, and waiting for things to be perfect just means missing out.

We have moments where we wonder if we should do something. It's natural to ask if now is the right time to chase a dream or make a change. But instead of reasons to wait, what if we asked, "Why not now?"

The more you question 'why now', the more excuses you find to delay.

When you stop making excuses and start working on your dreams, it's like pushing a snowball downhill – it gets easier and faster. Putting things off because of 'why now' leads to doubt and delays.

By saying, 'Why not now?' you become stronger and better at handling change. Instead of dwelling on reasons to wait, you find solutions and take action.

So, why not make this change today? Why not take a leap and see what happens? There's a whole world of possibilities waiting!

The Million-Dollar Question

We've all seen the before-and-after pictures: someone transformed from a couch potato to a fitness enthusiast, flabby to fit. These dramatic changes inspire us but leave us with a nagging question – how? The key to lasting change lies in a quiet corner of your mind: your mindset.

A temporary diet won't transform you if your core beliefs and motivations haven't shifted.

To cultivate vibrant blooms and flourishing vegetables, you wouldn't simply sprinkle seeds and hope for the best. You'd need fertile soil, consistent watering, and nurturing sunlight. Transforming your body requires a shift in how you think about yourself and your health.

Many people approach health with a seed of self-doubt already planted. "I'm not strong enough," or "I'll never look like that" are these little voices that hold you back. This negativity creates a barren mental landscape where healthy habits struggle to take root.

Social media bombards us with images of 'perfection', leading to the painful thorns of comparison. You see sculpted physiques and flawless complexions, and your own bodies suddenly feel inadequate. This constant comparison game fuels the fire of self-doubt, making positive change seem impossible.

The million-dollar question isn't 'What diet should I follow?' but rather 'Who do I need to be to stick with a healthy lifestyle?' Millions chase the perfect diet year after year, believing it's the magic bullet to weight loss. However, the real secret lies within – it's cultivating the mindset and habits that make healthy choices a natural extension of who you are. A temporary diet won't transform you if your core beliefs and motivations haven't shifted.

It's Not a One-Stop Shop

I meet a lot of folks these days, all fired up about getting ripped fast. They want a magic formula, a secret handshake to six-pack abs. The idea of building long-term health just doesn't seem to click. It's all about the immediate results, the quick fix.

Maybe you've heard the phrase, "Eat, drink, and be merry?" Well, these folks are looking for the 'eat, drink, and have rock-hard abs' version. They want the shortcut, the one-size-fits-all answer to unlocking incredible health.

There's no magic trick; it's all about who you become on the journey. Don't get me wrong, a strong core is fantastic! But true health is so much more.

It's about feeling energised, confident, and ready to tackle life's adventures.

So, why do so many people get caught up in this 'get ripped quick' mentality? It's easy. It feeds on that instant gratification culture we live in. We see those chiselled bodies on social media, and we want it – now. But that kind of thinking sets you up for disappointment.

Getting healthy takes consistent effort and learning about what works for your body. You wouldn't expect to train for a few days and suddenly be an Olympic athlete. So why chase that unrealistic ideal when it comes to your health? It's about progress, not perfection.

Now, I'm not saying you won't see changes along the way. You will! But they won't happen overnight. You will notice feeling less sluggish after a week of healthier eating. A month into a new workout routine, you'll feel those muscles getting stronger. Celebrate those milestones! They're proof that your hard work is paying off.

Quick fixes fade. True health is about building good habits, making smart choices, and becoming the best version of yourself. It's about feeling good, being strong, and having the energy to chase your dreams.

So, to those folks looking for the magic pill to health – I wish you good luck. You're going to need it.

Good and Bad

Life is a series of events that unfolds in mysterious ways. People label these events as either good or bad. A happy day feels good, a sad day feels bad. Sometimes, pieces seem to fit together perfectly. Other times, they don't seem to make sense. But is there really such a thing as good or bad? Or is it just the right thing happening at the right time?

The right thing happens at the right time, even if it doesn't feel right in the moment.

There are no labels like good or bad in life. Every event, every experience, every feeling happens for a reason at just the right time.

What seems 'bad' is merely the right thing happening when it should. Tough moments may feel awful. But it's a lesson you need to learn, a path you need to take. It will lead you to something better, something you couldn't have imagined before.

On the flip side, what we call 'good' is just the right thing at the right time. A joyful moment, a happy memory - it's perfect for that exact point in your journey. It might not last forever, but it's the right feeling for that moment. Every piece, no matter how it looks, has its place. And the whole picture, when it's complete, is beautiful.

You v/s Yesterday

Stop comparing your Chapter 3 to someone else's Chapter 10. This isn't a race against others; it's a climb against your own yesterday. Push yourself to be better than you were, stronger than you were. Let your competition be your own past self. Did you run a mile yesterday? Aim for a mile and a quarter today. Did you struggle with weight last week? Try it again this week. Success isn't about crushing everyone else. It's not about having a better body or being the strongest in the room. It's about becoming a better version of yourself, day by day.

> *The greatest victories are the ones we win over ourselves.*

Look in the mirror. Who do you see? Do you see someone stronger, healthier, and more confident than the person you were yesterday? That's the kind of competition that matters.

The greatest victories are the ones we win over ourselves. Forget about proving anything to anyone else. Play your own game, set your own goals, and celebrate each step up your personal mountain.

Find Your Finish Line

You hop in your car and start driving without a destination in mind. You just hit the road. Where will you end up? Somewhere, sure. But is it where you truly want to be? Probably not.

A journey can be full of growth, learning, and beautiful moments, but the destination provides the meaning for those experiences.

The journey can be beautiful, but the destination gives it purpose. It turns random actions into determined, meaningful steps. So, get clear on what you want. If you don't know where you're headed, it's just a long ride to nowhere. It's like reading a book without an ending. Sure, the story is good, but it's incomplete.

With a clear goal, every step you take has meaning. Every small victory pushes you closer to where you truly want to be. Never lose sight of where you're going. You're not just wandering; you're on a mission.

Earn Your Slice of Success

Everyone wants the good stuff, but no one wants to put in the work. It's kind of like that saying: "Everyone wants to go to heaven, but nobody wants to die."

When you finally hold that dream in your hand, you'll know exactly how much you deserve it.

Deep down, we all crave the best things in life – success, happiness, and that feeling of accomplishment. But those things rarely fall into our lap. It's like a delicious cake – you wouldn't just expect it to appear on your plate, right? You gotta mix the batter, bake it, and frost it!

Don't be discouraged if effort feels necessary. Every athlete trains, and every artist practices. The journey itself is where the magic happens. It's the struggles, the practice, the late nights that turn us into the people we're meant to be. So, roll up your sleeves, get ready to mix things up, and bake yourself a life you'll truly love. Because the feeling of accomplishment after reaching a goal is pure magic, when you finally hold that dream in your hand, you'll know exactly how much you deserve it.

People fear losing what they have more than they are excited about gaining what they want.

My friend was really worried about his son. The boy wasn't doing well at school. He failed an exam, which made my friend very upset. In an attempt to motivate him, my friend promised his son, "If you get good grades, I'll give you an extra $100 in pocket money." Sadly, the son still did not improve, and my friend was left wondering what to do next.

The thought of losing something makes us appreciate it more and work harder to keep it.

He shared his concerns with me. He asked, "What should I do with this boy?" I said, "Maybe try something different."

"What do you mean?" he asked.

"Well," I replied, "People are usually more afraid of losing what they already have than they are excited to gain something new." You tried to encourage him by giving him more money. This time, try reducing his pocket money if he doesn't improve. Sometimes, people only understand the value of something when they are about to lose it.

I didn't suggest this out of any ill will towards his son. I just wanted to help my friend find a way to motivate his son.

People don't take care of their health until they feel it's slipping away. You don't value it when you're healthy, but you realise its importance when you lose it.

The Final Countdown

Life is full of busy moments. We rush around, thinking every little thing is important. We wake up, go to work, stress about money, and argue with loved ones over silly things. Lost in screens, we forget what truly matters.

In life's final moments, health, love, and joy are what truly matter.

But when lying on a stretcher, fighting for your last breath, everything changes. The dim hospital lights flicker above, and the soft, steady beep of the machine contrasts sharply with the chaos in your mind. Fear grips your chest tighter. Suddenly, all those meetings, texts, and plans seem insignificant. The only thing that matters is survival. Every breath becomes precious, and every heartbeat feels like a countdown. In that moment, you wish for more time, more laughter, and more love. It's terrifying to realise how we let life slip by, filled with distractions.

Here on the stretcher, fighting desperately, you understand what truly matters. But it feels like a cruel joke, learning this lesson when time is almost gone. And that is the scariest realisation of all.

Alive but Not Living

If you feel your life is meaningless, it's up to you to determine its meaning.

Being alive is more than just breathing. It's about being full of energy and having the power to chase your dreams. When you are truly alive, you feel happy and satisfied. Life is about living big, not just getting by. Look for joy and meaning in every day. Living comes from pursuing what matters to you. Breathing keeps you physically present, but true aliveness comes from the heart and soul. It's about grabbing chances and loving moments. Live with passion and purpose. Don't just exist; make sure you are really living. Merely existing isn't enough; you need to thrive and truly enjoy all that life offers. As long as you're *alive*, you enjoy your life.

Live Free

Remember the lessons, but not the pain.

If you want a happy and healthy life, don't hold onto hate. Hate is like a heavy chain around your heart. It keeps you stuck in the past and blocks your happiness. Even if you let go of someone or something, if you still hate, it stays in your heart. If you want to forget something or someone, never hate it. Everything and everyone that you hate is engraved upon your heart; you can let go of something, or you can forget someone, but you cannot hate. Enjoy life by living without hate and let yourself truly be free.

I Don't Care

To achieve your dreams, ignite the fire of passion within you, and passion begins with care. To have passion, you must first care. You need to care to have passion. If you say you don't care, you don't have passion. You must care whether you win or lose. You must care if you fail, and you must care if you haven't achieved what you were supposed to by now. Because if you don't care, let me tell you, it's not going to happen. So, don't say, "I don't care."

If you don't care, you won't learn from the struggles.

If you don't care, you'll miss the opportunities.

If you don't care, you'll settle for mediocrity.

If you don't care, you won't find passion in the work.

If you don't care, you'll lack the discipline.

If you don't care, you'll fail to see your potential.

If you don't care, you'll stop trying when it gets hard.

You gotta *care* about your growth.

You gotta *care* about your relationships.

You gotta *care* about your mindset.

You gotta *care* about making a difference.

You gotta *care* about your priorities.

You gotta *care* about your time.

You gotta *care* about your dreams and aspirations.

You gotta *care* about your well-being.

You gotta *care* about the effort you put in.

You gotta *care* about the values you uphold.

You gotta *care* about how you treat yourself and others.

You gotta *care* about setting a good example.

One Last Thing to Remember

Life can be quite challenging, and it often feels like there just aren't enough hours in the day. That's why I choose to finish my workout first thing when I wake up. It sets a positive tone for the day. Even if things get busy and plans change, I know I've already accomplished something important. It frees up the rest of my day. I don't have to worry about squeezing in a workout.

I believe in starting the day with a victory. No matter how small, it helps to set the right mood. So, even when the day doesn't go as planned, I have achieved something that's just for me. I'm making a promise to myself that today is mine, and I will make the most out of it.

Making the choice to prioritize your health and well-being is a commitment to yourself, a moment of peace before diving into the day. And in that commitment, you'll find strength and joy.

Yes, it is hard, but that's the point. If you want to get things done, you have to be willing to do the hard things. If you want to win, you have to do what others aren't doing.

Do the uncomfortable until it becomes comfortable.

There are 4 kinds of people: those who fail, those who lose, those who want to win, and those who actually win (winners). Giving up makes you a loser, and you lose the chance to experience victory. If you fail but continue trying, you still have opportunities to win. Wanting to win and persisting in your efforts ultimately makes you a winner.

In life, sometimes you have to make choices. Big choices or little ones, each asks a whispery question - yes, or no? Every day, you get to pick 'yes' or 'no' and every 'yes' and 'no' shapes your day.It's about priority. When something truly matters to you, you'll find the time and energy to make it happen. You'll be willing to make adjustments to fit it in. But if something isn't important to you, you'll come up with excuses and find reasons to avoid it. You'll try to convince yourself why you can't do it.

You avoid doing things not because you can't do them. *You can, but you don't want to. If you really want to, you can.*

Have you figured it out yet? The sole purpose of your life is to be happy. And health is power, the power to live a life that makes you happy.

The second-best advice I can give you is to make friends, make time, make money, and make a life you're proud of. Make everything except excuses.

I wasn't always the person I am today. I used to be a mess. I wasn't the best student and wasn't a good son, brother, or husband. I made a lot of mistakes, and I always felt lost. For a long time, I blamed everyone else for my problems. It was always someone else's fault or the circumstances around me that were to blame.

But it all changed when I realised I needed to look inside myself first. I understood that if I wanted my life to get better, I had to change myself. I had to stop blaming others and take responsibility for my actions and situation.

I discovered that loving myself was the first step towards being loved and respected by others. To live a happy, healthy and joyful life, I knew I had to work on myself. I learned that showing gratitude helped me see the positives in everything around me. It shifted my perspective and made me appreciate the little things in life.

I realised that my health is the one thing that keeps me going and gives me the strength to achieve my goals, follow my passion, and live my purpose.

Life isn't perfect, but it's brighter and more fulfilling than ever before.

Thank you for taking the time to read the book. I am truly grateful. I hope you found something meaningful, and I hope my words inspire you to make positive changes in your life.

About the Author

Shah Emran, known publicly as just Shah, is an author whose work engages readers through insightful explorations of real-world topics. He believes that the world needs more people passionate about making a positive impact on their own lives and the world around them.

Despite holding a master's degree, Shah values life lessons over formal education. He emphasises the importance of continuous learning and personal growth rather than just earning degrees.

Shah is deeply convinced that everyone has a purpose in life—a guiding force. His purpose: To help people achieve strength in both body and mind. His mission is to inspire and empower people around the world, encouraging them to find and pursue their own unique purpose.

Through his writing and personal philosophy, Shah strives to motivate people to make positive changes, cultivate resilience, and live fulfilling lives.